Body Building

The Definitive Manual On Bodybuilding Nutrition And Supplements For Optimal Muscle Growth Acceleration

(Efficient Methodologies And App............ .... .ιγsique
Enhancement In Males Above 50 Years Of Age)

Larry Birch

TABLE OF CONTENT

Introduction

This book offers verified methods and approaches for effectively enhancing muscle development and reducing body fat through the implementation of dietary adjustments and supplementary practices.

Undoubtedly, we must acknowledge that beauty holds a revered status in contemporary society. For women, the desired attributes often include delicate, fair complexion and an hourglass figure, while men tend to strive for a lean, muscular physique and an assertive, rough and masculine appearance. Such is the significance of this elusive concept in the context of our contemporary existence, that numerous misconceptions and inaccurate narratives have emerged, claiming to guide and assist us in its pursuit. Frequently, we become so engrossed in our pursuit of enhancing our appearance that we readily embrace these misleading assertions.

An enduring fallacy prevailing in the realm of beauty and physical fitness revolves around the notion that in order to increase muscle mass, one must engage in rigorous weightlifting exercises at a gym and concurrently consume copious amounts of protein. Only the minimum level of carbohydrate consumption necessary for sustaining adequate energy levels is prescribed.

However, it is a fact that consuming an ample and appropriate diet is merely one of the strategies we can employ to expedite the process of muscle development. Indeed, dating back to the era of ancient Greece, individuals involved in athletic endeavors and strenuous physical activities have been advised to adopt a traditional dietary approach that is equally ancient. This approach entails the consumption of higher quantities of meat and wine compared to the typical diet. Supplements have historically been employed to fulfill a similar purpose, as observed in the practices of various cultures' strongmen. These individuals utilized herbal concoctions and comparable substances as aids to augment their energy, physical abilities, and endurance.

Thank you once again for taking the time to download this book. It is my sincerest hope that you derive great enjoyment from it.

We kindly invite you to explore our official website, Wilson Press.
http://wilsonpressbooks.com

The primary objective of this document is to furnish precise and dependable information pertaining to the subject matter and concern addressed. The published material is marketed on the premise that the publisher is not obligated to provide accounting or official authorized services, or any other services that require specific qualifications. If advice of a legal or professional nature is deemed necessary, it is recommended to engage the services of a skilled practitioner in the respective field.

- As per an accepted and approved Declaration of Principles, endorsed equally by both a Committee of the American Bar Association and a Committee of Publishers and Associations.

5

Arnold Schwarzenegger, widely regarded as the preeminent bodybuilder of his era, espoused the principles of employing fundamental compound movements, incorporating substantial weights, implementing high-intensity training techniques, and employing high volume workouts.

If one aspires to emulate the training regimen of esteemed figures such as Arnold and other renowned bodybuilders, it is advisable to adhere to this prescribed training strategy.

Engaging in strength training: utilizing heavy loads and employing correct form while exercising leads to an increase in muscle size and strength. In this training session, it is imperative that you select a weight of sufficient heaviness, rendering it extremely difficult for you to lift, to the point where your muscles are incapable of performing more than 8 repetitions.

Emphasizing Volume: Opt for a significant number of sets to train the desired muscle group - typically, the preferred and highly effective approach by esteemed bodybuilders entails performing around 20 to 30 sets for each muscle group.

⬜ Reduce utilization of machines and isolation exercises: Compound weightlifting exercises such as parallel bar dips and barbell/dumbbell shoulder press, pull ups, deadlifts, squats, barbell and dumbbell shrugs, cable lat pull downs, and cable seated rows are optimal movements for developing a highly resilient physique. Reduce the utilization of machine and isolation exercises as their efficacy tends to be relatively low.

Engage in experimentation: alter your grips, foot stance, and angles marginally to enhance force exertion and muscle stretching, akin to Arnold Schwarzenegger's approach.

⬚ Embrace positive behaviors: Make a conscious effort to choose nutritious foods and steer clear of unhealthy options lacking in nutritional value. Prioritize sufficient rest and enhance your social interactions, as these endeavors can help cultivate popularity and foster feelings of self-assurance and self-worth.

By exercising within a designated repetition range, you can effectively enhance the development of robust and resilient muscles within a relatively condensed timeframe. According to esteemed and accomplished bodybuilders such as Arnold Schwarzenegger, engaging in a challenging set of 6-8 repetitions is equally demanding compared to performing a strenuous set of 20 repetitions using a lighter weight. Engaging in 20 repetitions using significantly lighter weights does not provide a satisfactory means of attaining the muscle growth achievable through the utilization of heavier weights and a range of 6-8 repetitions.

If you are engaged in the pursuit of muscle development, it is to be expected that you are already aware that solely engaging in exercise is not adequate. The diet regimen also holds significant importance. Adopting a dietary regimen akin to that of body builders has been observed to aid in achieving a toned physique and shedding surplus weight, particularly when accompanied by an appropriate exercise regimen. The fundamental concept entails consuming a diet abundant in protein and fiber, while minimizing the intake of carbohydrates and fat. This diet also incorporates more frequent meal consumption.

Upon examination of the dietary regimens followed by renowned bodybuilders, one will discern that each adheres to distinct meal plans involving disparate food compositions, meal timings, and macronutrient ratios. Nevertheless, they all remain steadfast in adhering to overarching fundamental principles. Let us examine the dietary choices made by certain celebrities.

Arnold Schwarzenegger

The septuple winner of Mr. Olympia would primarily focus on consuming unprocessed, organic nourishment and abstaining from extensively manufactured food items. Several of the principles he proposed are:

Consume 5-6 smaller meals daily

It is recommended to consume carbohydrates within a 30-minute timeframe following physical activity.

Ensure a daily intake of 30 to 50 grams of proteins per meal.

One should not refrain from consuming saturated fat owing to its potential to elevate hormonal levels.

Kindly restrict your daily egg consumption to a maximum of 3 eggs.

Swap out beef and pork in favor of poultry and fish

⬚ Avoid the consumption of sugar as it contains empty calories. Instead, opt for vegetables and fruits to obtain carbohydrates.

Employ dietary supplements and protein shakes in order to attain the essential daily requirement of protein.

Ronnie Coleman

Coleman has undergone significant transformations in the past and has shared his daily dietary regimen for physique enhancement on a few occasions. One variant comprises of cheese grits, along with poultry, egg white, and beef.

Furthermore, he has exhibited his dietary habits in each of his workout videos. In a single video recording, he consumes a substantial amount of hamburger with copious amounts of barbecue sauce on all his food items and indulges in a combination of Sprite and grape juice, which are not the most conventional dietary choices in terms of maintaining a clean eating regimen.

Some of the stipulations comprise consuming 2 grams of protein per pound of body weight (equivalent to 600 grams daily and 100 grams per meal.) He partakes in six meals per day, with his primary protein sources being chicken, steak, and turkey.

Jay Cutler

His daily calorie target is nearly 4,700, with a focus on maintaining a macronutrient ratio of approximately 40% protein, 40% carbohydrates, and 20% fat. Cutler also incorporates a substantial amount of poultry and brown rice into his diet. In addition, he devotes a significant portion of his day, approximately 5-6 hours, to food preparation and eating. The proposed time allocation per day is undeniably excessive and poses a daunting level of complexity when performed consistently, surpassing the difficulty of any physical exercise regimen.

Jay also experiences nocturnal awakenings to consume additional food, attributing this behavior to the purported loss of around 10 pounds during his sleeping hours. The majority of his carbohydrate intake is derived from simple carbohydrates, as he claims that his size diminishes when consuming complex carbohydrates.

A few of his previous dietary regimes incorporated ample portions of oats and sweet potatoes, but it seems that his present regimen has substituted these with white and brown rice. He ingests an estimated amount of 2 pounds of chicken and beef on a daily basis, along with a preference for consuming 2 servings of egg white accompanied by Ezekiel toast each morning.

Dorian Yates

Yates recommends a protein intake of 1-1.5 grams per pound of body weight, and advises doubling that amount for carbohydrate consumption.

Historically, the suggested fat intake has been estimated to be approximately one-third of the recommended protein consumption. An individual ingesting 300 grams of proteins would be receiving 600 grams of carbohydrates and 100 grams of fats, resulting in a cumulative caloric intake of 4500 calories.

Choosing the Right Diet

In order to develop a preliminary dietary regimen, it is imperative to ascertain your current status. It is imperative to ascertain an effective methodology to accurately monitor your weight and body fat composition. The sole consideration of weight, as well as the exclusive focus on body fat percentage, do not offer a comprehensive assessment of one's progress. However, when these two elements are combined, they can provide a reasonably precise method for tracking both fat mass and body mass.

If, regrettably, one fails to diligently monitor their progress, it will certainly prove to be arduous to effect any alterations in the designated dietary regimen, ascertaining the nature of the weight gained - be it muscle or fat - becomes a formidable task.

23 Effective Training Strategies to Enhance Performance, Promote Muscle Growth, Facilitate Fat Loss, Enhance Strength, and Achieve Significant Physique Development

Tip 1: Compound Movements

If you desire to maximize your return on investment, compound movements present an optimal solution. Engaging in isolation exercises such as bicep curls, tricep pulldowns, and calf raises, among others. Stimulation of those specific muscles will occur through isolated movements, whereas compound exercises engage multiple muscle groups simultaneously, triggering a substantial surge of growth hormone and facilitating the breakdown of numerous muscle fibers concurrently.

Tip 2: The Deadlift

The deadlift, considered the pinnacle of back exercises, holds significant importance in the arsenal of a bodybuilder, as it effectively engages not only the entirety of the back muscles but also targets the hamstrings. Ensure that you exercise great attention to detail in perfecting your form as you learn this particular movement. I have observed numerous individuals engaging in fitness activities, and I have found it necessary to provide guidance on their technique. Persisting with incorrect form could potentially lead to severe spinal complications in the future. It is evident that verbally describing the deadlift would pose challenges; hence, I recommend referring to a concise instructional video by renowned weightlifting expert, Elliott Hulse. Mr. Hulse possesses extensive experience in the field of weightlifting, including a professional strongman career, rendering him a highly credible authority on the subject matter.

Recommendation 3: The Clean and Press

This compound movement effectively targets both the muscles in the legs and the shoulder region, resulting in a highly beneficial exercise. Once again, commence with a minimal weight and gradually progress to avoid the risk of injury and forfeiting the progress you have made at the gym.

Tip number four: The incline press

The flat barbell bench press proves to be highly effective. It is considered as a cornerstone exercise for chest development and concurrently targets the anterior deltoids and triceps. Nevertheless, incorporating the incline press into your workout routine will result in a considerably more visually appealing pectoral region. It enhances the development of the pectoralis major muscles, resulting in a more robust and masculine aesthetic. This exercise is executed by following the same technique as the bench press, but with the bench inclined at approximately a 45-degree angle. I recommend that you experiment with different bench angles to determine which ones are most effective for you.

Additional suggestion: "An additional valuable suggestion: For those interested, it is advantageous to review archived footage of Arnold Schwarzenegger engaging in training sessions. Notably, in the incline press exercise, Schwarzenegger adopts a remarkably broad grip." Based on my personal observations, this technique enables a comprehensive extension of the upper pectoral muscles, thereby ensuring that the pectoral muscles bear a significant portion of the load as opposed to the triceps.

Point 5: Regulating your intervals of rest

If your objective is to enhance muscular strength, it is advisable to maintain lengthier periods of rest. A duration ranging between 3-5 minutes would be highly satisfactory. Should you require additional time for rest, it is advisable to extend the duration of your rest periods. To enhance muscular development, I suggest maintaining rest periods of no more than 90 seconds (preferably falling within the 60-90 seconds range). This intervention is designed to specifically enhance the production of growth hormone in your body and stimulate hypertrophy.

I have the capability to delve into the comprehensive details of the process, elucidate the intricate scientific terminology, and elaborate on the subject matter extensively. Nevertheless, I must acknowledge that the counsel I received derives from esteemed figures in the online fitness community, namely Elliott Hulse and Brandon Carter, renowned luminaries in the field. If you desire evidence that is considered reliable, I invite you to peruse their pages.

Recommendation 6: Adhere to the use of unfettered weights

From a personal standpoint, I must admit that this is a matter of subjective inclination. I have reservations regarding the utilization of machinery. When operating the machines, one does not engage the various small stabilizer muscles essential for executing other bodily functional movements. This implies that while you may possess the ability to execute significant bench press weight on the smith machine, the resultant strength may not effectively translate to other exercises due to insufficient development of your stabilizer muscles.

While machines can certainly serve a purpose, it is advisable to prioritize the utilization of predominantly free weights in one's fitness regimen. Incorporating free weights into your fitness routine will engage and strengthen your stabilizer muscles. Additionally, it will enhance your core strength and fortify your structural integrity, resulting in enhanced performance in your other exercises.

Tip 7: Pre Exhaustion

Suppose you are engaged in a bench press exercise. This marks the inaugural set of your workout as you focus on training your pectoral muscles during today's session. The initial two sets are executed quite effectively, resulting in a noticeable contraction in the triceps and chest muscles, generating a pleasantly satisfying sensation. As the third set approaches, one can sense the triceps becoming fatigued while the chest remains determined. However, as the fourth set ensues, further repetitions become unattainable due to the excessive strain on the triceps, despite the lingering sensation that the chest could complete a few more repetitions.

This is the context in which the pre-exhaustion method becomes relevant. The implementation of the pre-exhaustion technique enables the pre-fatiguing of a particular muscle group through an isolation exercise, followed by the execution of a compound movement targeting the same muscle group. Let us consider an instance where, prior to engaging in the bench press exercise, one can perform a set of chest flys to effectively pre-exhaust the targeted muscle. You will experience a slight increase in cardiovascular activity within the chest area, ensuring that when transitioning to the bench press exercise, both the triceps and chest muscles will reach a point of muscle fatigue simultaneously, preventing premature triceps exhaustion prior to achieving optimal chest stimulation.

When attempting this technique, it is important to bear in mind that you should select an isolation exercise that complements the compound movement. For instance, one could consider incorporating chest flys in conjunction with bench press, lateral raises alongside military press, and leg curls in combination with squats.

"Step 8: Developing Substantial Upper Limbs

It is a prevailing belief among individuals who are new to the realm of bodybuilding that performing a substantial quantity of bicep curls is the key to achieving significant arm muscle development, correct? I intend to elucidate that the form of physical activity being referred to is commonly portrayed in motion pictures and televised productions, mainly depicting individuals engaged in exercise, particularly the exercise known as the dumbbell bicep curl.

I will confide a confidential piece of information to you. Your upper limb consists of a composition where the tricep comprises two parts and the bicep accounts for one part. This implies that if one desires to significantly increase the size of their arms, the most effective approach would be to prioritize the development of their triceps muscles. There are numerous methods through which one may develop their triceps; notable among them involves engaging in pressing exercises such as the bench press, incline press, shoulder press, and Pushups, as these movements elicit pronounced triceps contraction. If you are seeking effective isolation exercises, both the dumbbell skull crushers and the close grip bench press are commendable options.

Step 9: Achieving the V-Taper Physique

The V-shaped physique is characterized by well-developed, broad shoulders and a tapered waistline in males. It exhibits a visually appealing aesthetic, and is favored by women. To the best of my knowledge, there are currently no exercise regimens available that specifically target waist reduction. However, it is possible to engage in exercises that can effectively enhance shoulder broadness. Specifically, engaging in military presses and lateral raises will facilitate the development and fortification of the deltoid muscles located on the sides of your shoulders, resulting in the desired aesthetically pleasing V-shaped appearance.

Tip 10: Isolation movements

As previously mentioned, it is advisable to primarily focus on incorporating compound exercises into your workout routine. These exercises have the ability to engage a greater number of muscle fibers and induce a more substantial release of growth hormone. Nevertheless, should you possess a few particularly underdeveloped muscle groups (which is common for everyone), it is permissible to incorporate a few specific sets to emphasize those areas of weakness. Specifically focusing on my calves, I allocate three sessions per week to enhance their development. Towards the conclusion of my workout routine, I engage in targeted isolation exercises for my calves.

Step 11: Enhancing Back Thickness Development

A well-developed dorsal musculature is indicative of significant traits in a male individual. Not only do women appreciate well-developed shoulders with prominent, three-dimensional contours, but the back also plays a critical role in enhancing functional strength. In order to enhance the muscle thickness of your back, it will be necessary to perform a significant number of row exercises. This entails executing barbell rows (with appropriate technique), dumbbell rows, and inverted bodyweight rows. Please ensure that you maintain proper elbow positioning, keeping them calmly close to your body, and consciously engage your back muscles while performing the exercise. A significant number of individuals mistakenly believe that they are exerting effort, but in reality, they are not effectively doing so. Make sure to pull through with your elbows and squeeze the back together, hold for 1-2 seconds, then release.

Tip 12: Supersets

For those among you who are unfamiliar, a superset entails completing a singular set of one exercise directly followed by a set of another exercise. The superset may encompass a variety of options, encompassing either the targeting of similar muscle groups or the engagement of opposing muscle groups. Supersets effectively reduce the duration of your workout while simultaneously enhancing its intensity.

I engage in specific supersets that effectively target the identical muscle groups, including close grip upright rows and elbow-bent lateral raises. Both of these exercises primarily focus on the trapezius muscles and provide a considerable hypertrophic response to this specific muscle group. Additionally, there are supersets that specifically focus on working opposing muscle groups. Arnold demonstrated a strong endorsement for incorporating chest/back supersets into his workout regimen. He states that the sensation of muscular engorgement achieved by performing a series on the incline press directly followed by a sequence of chin-ups is truly exemplary.

Tip 13: Deload week

I am a staunch proponent of this particular matter. Resistance training places significant strain on the body, necessitating the periodic allocation of 5-7 days of rest every 3-4 months in order to promote optimal physical recovery. Now, it is imperative to ensure that you engage in rigorous and sustained training, as a mere attendance of three gym sessions in one week does not suffice to claim diligent effort. It is now the appropriate period for a week of deloading. Regrettably, my friend, that approach does not suffice. Engage in rigorous training for a period of 3-4 months, followed by a subsequent week-long hiatus from your training routine.

Chapter 14: A Comparison Between Dumbbells and Barbell

Determining the appropriate choice between dumbbells and barbells can be rather perplexing, given the myriad of considerations to take into account. Each possesses its own set of strengths and weaknesses. Fundamentally, the employment of a barbell enables a more efficient means of exerting higher levels of weight to target and stimulate the muscles, as it typically allows for greater lifting capacities compared to a set of dumbbells. Nevertheless, dumbbells have a propensity for remedying muscular imbalances as well as facilitating a more profound and controlled elongation during exercises. I would recommend incorporating both of these methods into your exercise regimen.

Guideline 15: Engage in exercises that promote muscle growth

Indeed, engaging in displays of physical prowess serves a purpose beyond mere vanity. Additionally, engaging in flexing exercises enhances the synergy between your mind and muscles, augmenting the blood flow directed towards the targeted muscle group. Considering that Arnold incorporated this practice into the conclusion of his workout routine, it would be prudent to explore any approach endorsed by Arnold with a sense of credibility.

Tip 16: Drop sets

Ooh man. If you have yet to experience this, prepare for an incredibly rewarding encounter. Dropping sets entails executing a maximum number of repetitions on a given exercise, subsequently reducing the weight by approximately 20%, and proceeding to perform another set with a maximum number of repetitions. This exercise effectively fatigues and stimulates the muscles, leading to a pronounced muscle pump. I would encourage you to test it with the bench press apparatus and evaluate your satisfaction. Select an appropriate amount of weight that allows you to perform only 5 repetitions, subsequently reduce the weight by removing a few plates, and proceed to perform an additional set of 5 repetitions.

Recommendation 17: Ensure that the major muscle groups undergo training at least once weekly.

Yes, even legs folks. One cannot exhibit a protruding chest to attract women when accompanied by excessively thin legs. Ensure that you incorporate a comprehensive strength training regimen that includes an intensive session for each of the primary muscle groups, namely the legs, chest, back, and shoulders.

Recommendation 18: Incorporate Cardiovascular Training While Striving for Muscle Growth

Individuals often exhibit apprehension towards engaging in cardiovascular exercise while pursuing muscle development. Believing that a single hour of sustained cardiovascular exercise will inexplicably result in the complete depletion of muscle gains and strength. This is the most absurd statement I have ever come across. Provided that you maintain a sufficient intake of calories, you will be adequately sustained. I engage in steady-state, low-intensity, high-volume cardio exercises on an empty stomach to effectively maintain a low level of body fat, which aligns with my personal regimen.

Recommendation 19: Incorporating Chest Flys to Enhance Muscle Development

Indeed, the bench press and incline press exercises are highly effective for eliciting substantial muscular development in the pectoral region. Nevertheless, the chest fly is capable of efficiently supplying ample blood to the muscles without exerting excessive strain on the triceps or front deltoids. By observing videos of Arnold performing chest flys with precision, where he engages the pectoral muscles deeply and accentuates their contraction at the apex of the movement, one can ascertain that this technique fosters excellent chest stimulation and contributes significantly to chest development.

Tips 20: Supplements

Supplements are great. However, they are solely that and nothing more. A supplement. Partial nourishment, these supplements are intended to complement and enhance the nutritional needs of your body. Whey protein and creatine are widely regarded as the most effective choices for enhancing muscle development. That's it. Abstain from using pre-workout supplements and elaborate fat burners; instead, by solely relying on these two, you will effectively cultivate lean muscle mass.

Tips 21: Novice individuals - there is no need for concern regarding Delayed Onset Muscle Soreness (DOMS).

Holy shit. I distinctly recall the initial instance when I engaged in weightlifting, subsequently experiencing notable discomfort in my calf muscles for a duration of approximately five days. And the discomfort intensified during that period. If one experiences delayed onset muscle soreness, there is no need to be concerned. Engaging in light-hearted strolls resembling the gait of a pigeon for a duration of approximately one week. You witnessed it here, newcomers. It is entirely expected and typical to experience significant muscle soreness following your initial exercise session.

Key Recommendation 22: Implement Public Relations (PR) for Each Exercise Session

I also encounter this issue. In my every workout session, my goal is to attain a new personal record. However, this approach exerts considerable strain on both the mental and physical aspects of my being. Simply entering the gym and engaging in physical activity already positions you as a victor; any subsequent achievements are merely supplementary. Not every exercise session necessitates achieving a personal record.

Principle 23: Prioritizing Form over Weight

In the past, I held the belief that augmenting one's weight bestowed a sense of "coolness." Therefore, you have the potential to personify the epitome of strength and become renowned as the individual who effortlessly conquers the most formidable weights at the gym.

Allow me to express that removing one's ego will lead to significant and meaningful progress. There exist alternative methods to enhance the exercise's intensity without augmenting the weight, and a viable approach in achieving this is through proper form.

When you exhibit proper form, the intended musculature is effectively activated. When one engages in weightlifting driven by ego, it can inadvertently involve additional muscle groups that were not intended to be focused upon. As a case in point, consider the scenario where one engages in the bench press exercise while attempting to, quite literally, bear more weight than within their capacity. In this situation, it is evident that a larger portion of the weight load will be transmitted to the anterior deltoid muscles rather than the pectoral muscles. You might be under the impression that you are effectively targeting your chest muscles by lifting heavy weights, but in reality, you are primarily engaging your front deltoids and not placing enough emphasis on your chest.

Prioritize the completion of the form before proceeding with other tasks. Deliberately engage the muscle during each exercise, and subsequently focus on gradually augmenting the resistance.

Reduce adipose tissue and maintain lean muscle mass through a daily five-minute regimen.

By adhering to a specific training regimen for a duration of five minutes daily, five days a week, one can efficiently reduce body fat while maintaining muscle mass.

The straightforward technique you are about to acquire will...

Attain a well-defined physique, while preserving muscle mass.

Promote the reduction of fat while preserving lean muscle and tissue mass.

Tone and sculpt your buttocks. (A gentleman's posterior is the aspect that garners the attention of the majority of women.)

It is understandable if one were to believe that extensive periods of aerobic exercise are necessary. This is what is widely regarded as the method to effectively reduce body fat. Nevertheless, appearances can be deceiving.

A widely held belief posits that simultaneous weight loss and muscle gain is an improbable endeavor. This holds true in the case of conventional prolonged aerobic sessions.

Extensive research has substantiated the notion that prolonged aerobic sessions metabolize body tissue as an energy source. This encompasses the musculature within your body. Furthermore, it does not effectively facilitate fat burning. These facts have been substantiated by numerous scientific studies.

The optimal approach to fat burning entails enhancing your metabolic rate.

The metabolic rate refers to the pace at which energy is expended by your body. This phenomenon is the reason behind the sustenance of a thin physique among specific individuals, despite their consumption of nutritionally inadequate foods and lack of physical activity. The metabolism is responsible for the combustion of adipose tissue. The key to effectively reducing fat while preserving muscle mass lies in enhancing metabolic activity.

How is that accomplished?
Fat is metabolized by your body's metabolic processes during periods of physical inactivity. Indeed, a significant reduction in adipose tissue oxidation occurs during physical activity. The crucial aspect in enhancing the rate of fat loss to its fullest extent lies in engaging in physical activity using a specific methodology.

What sort of physical activity do you engage in? Engage in high-intensity interval training. This phenomenon has been scientifically validated to facilitate a greater level of fat combustion in comparison to conventional aerobics. There is a substantial body of research supporting this assertion.

There exist numerous methods for engaging in interval training. Nevertheless, there is one method that proves to be particularly effective. You are only required to allocate five minutes of your time for this task. You perform this task on a regular basis from Monday to Friday. A period of two days is allocated for the purpose of recuperation.

How do you accomplish this? You merely ascend the stairs and subsequently descend on foot. You persist in engaging in this behavior for a duration of five minutes.

Through this approach, the intensity of the running component is significantly heightened compared to extended distance runs. This is due to the fact that during an extended duration, your speed will be significantly diminished. Hence, the physical activity will be considerably more moderate.

Due to the high intensity of stair running, five-minute sessions are sufficient. It requires a mere five minutes to enhance your metabolic rate for approximately twelve hours.

Alternative phrasing in a formal tone: "Additional forms of interval training, such as engaging in running, may be employed." Nevertheless, due to its relatively less vigorous nature as compared to stair running, a longer duration of sessions will be required to achieve equivalent results. Interval training requires a minimum duration of twenty minutes per session to achieve equivalent outcomes.

Ascending stairs proves to be the most optimal approach as it minimizes the time required to attain the utmost outcomes. That amounts to a total of twenty-five minutes per week, with a daily commitment of five minutes.

Does it work? You bet. I have received feedback from numerous individuals who have achieved weight loss through this method. They have experienced a greater reduction in weight compared to alternative approaches they have previously attempted.

It also provides an additional advantage. It displays noticeable efficacy in sculpting and toning your gluteal region, a feature which many women readily acknowledge as attractive in men. This is attributed to the elevated leg movement required to ascend staircases.

The plan is simple. Ascend the flight of stairs at a brisk pace, then descend using a measured gait. Please persist in carrying out this action for a duration of five minutes. Establish a timer to alleviate the need for frequent time checking.

Please ensure that this task is carried out on a regular basis, five days within each week. Take two days off. Your physical well-being will require a period of recuperation.

Initially, you may encounter challenges with this form of training, unless you are already in an exceptional physical condition. If you are initially unable to complete a five-minute duration, it is advised to complete as many minutes as you are capable of. You will soon discover that you will be capable of continuously performing stair running for the full duration of five minutes.

This encapsulates everything that is involved. Occasionally, the most effective approach is to embrace simplicity.

Chapter 2 - Initiating Proper Practices for Bodybuilding

One may commence an endeavor as soon as there exists a justification for undertaking it. What are your aspirations in the realm of bodybuilding? Please ensure that you consistently keep in mind the underlying purpose or motivation behind your pursuit of bodybuilding. It is imperative to establish specific objectives in order to maintain your engagement and fortify your determination. Similar to any endeavor or aspiration, it is often effortless to succumb to discouragement and abandon one's pursuits in the absence of visible advancements.

Females who commence their training for the first time exhibit equivalent levels of enthusiasm and impatience. They are eager to witness prompt outcomes. Nevertheless, if you aspire for your training to yield fruitful outcomes, there are factors that necessitate contemplation and deliberate pursuit.

One essential factor to bear in mind is the necessity of exerting diligent effort. Although an abundance of products and supplements claim to facilitate the attainment of the desired body mass, the majority of these assertions have proven to be unfounded. It is imperative that you acquire a meticulously structured training regimen that will effectively propel you towards the attainment of your objectives. You must exert self-control and adhere to your established regimen.

Another noteworthy aspect pertains to your dietary habits. It is crucial to ensure that your body receives adequate nutrition while engaging in weight training. Sufficient rest is also imperative. Develop a regimen that aligns with your aspirations in bodybuilding.

Third is the supplementation. Please be advised that neglecting proper nourishment, failing to adhere to a suitable regimen, and lacking discipline of the mind can potentially result in detrimental consequences to your organs.

In the subsequent chapters, a comprehensive account pertaining to the three pivotal aspects of bodybuilding, namely training, nutrition and supplements, shall be presented. Although it is a truism, knowledge holds great authority. Dedicate ample time to thoroughly studying and effectively integrating the knowledge you acquire in order to actively work towards the accomplishment of your objectives. You are entitled to attaining a physically alluring and robust physique through bodybuilding, and it is within your reach!

During the first block, encompassing a span of four weeks

It is advised to employ lighter weights during the initial two-week period. As you continue, you may advance to more substantial weights. Kindly refrain from exerting excessive effort in situations that may compromise your safety and comfort. Increase the load once you have gained a thorough comprehension of the movements and their proper sensation. "Presented below is an exemplar schedule:

Day 1

• Utilize a foam roller

• Perform 5 sets of Barbell Squats with one leg, completing 5 repetitions in each set.

• Complete three sets of barbell hip thrusts, with 12 repetitions in each set. • Perform three sets of barbell hip thrusts, with 12 reps in each set. • Execute three sets of barbell hip thrusts, with 12 repetitions per set. • Engage in three sets of barbell hip thrusts, completing 12 reps per set. • Undertake three sets of barbell hip thrusts, with 12 repetitions in each set.

• Box Jumps – Perform 20 repetitions, divided into multiple sets.

• Calf Press – Perform three sets of eight repetitions per set.

• Performing the Lying Leg Curl exercise for a total of 3 sets, with each set consisting of 12 repetitions.

• Vigorous Cardiovascular Exercise – 20 minutes

Day 2

• Perform the Push Up exercise for a total of 5 sets, with 5 repetitions per set.

• Dips – Perform 3 sets with 8 repetitions in each set.

• Medicine Ball Chest Pass - Perform 20 repetitions, dividing them into multiple sets.

• Cable Flye – Three sets with eight repetitions per set.

• Performing Lying Dumbbell Triceps Extensions – 3 sets (12 repetitions per set)

• Vigorous cardiovascular exercise - 20 minutes

Day 3

• Low intensity cardiovascular exercise - duration of 20 minutes.

Day 4

• Romanian Deadlift – Perform 5 sets, with 5 repetitions in each set.

• Bent-over Row – Three sets consisting of eight repetitions per set.

• Kettlebell Swings – Perform 20 repetitions, distributed across multiple sets.

• Latissimus Dorsi Pull-down Exercise – 3 sets (with 8 repetitions in each set)

• Perform the Incline Biceps Curl exercise with 3 sets, each set consisting of 12 repetitions.

• Vigorous Cardiovascular Exercise - 20-minute duration

Day 5

• The exercise known as the Dumbbell Press should be performed in a structured manner, with a total of five sets, each consisting of five repetitions.

• Perform three sets of eight repetitions for bottoms-up exercises.

• Perform 20 repetitions of Medicine Ball Throw Overhead, divided into multiple sets.

• Face Pull – Perform 3 sets consisting of 8 repetitions in each set.

• Perform three sets of planks, with 12 repetitions per set.

• Vigorous Cardiovascular Activity – 20 minutes • Intense Aerobic Exercise – 20 minutes • Rigorous Cardiorespiratory Training – 20 minutes

Days 6 and 7 - Scheduled period of rest

For the duration of Block 2, spanning Weeks 5 to 8

Modifying the principal motion will lead to advancements in your training. You will need to acquire additional lifting apparatus. The objective is to enhance the magnitude of your principal action on a weekly basis. Progress is imperative.

Day 1

• Perform 5 sets of front squats, with 5 repetitions per set.

• The exercise of choice is the Seated Leg Curl, to be performed in three sets, with each set consisting of eight repetitions.

• Perform 20 repetitions of box jumps, dividing them into multiple sets.

• Three sets of seated half-calf raises consisting of eight repetitions per set will be performed.

• Perform the Single-Leg Hip Thrust exercise in 3 sets, completing 8 repetitions per set.

• Leg Extensions – Perform 3 sets of 12 repetitions per set.

• Vigorous Cardiovascular Exercise – 20 minutes

Day 2

• Three sets of dumbbell bench press, with eight repetitions per set, will be performed.

• Perform the Medicine Ball Pass exercise for a total of 20 repetitions, with the sets being divided into smaller increments.

• Dip exercise - 3 sets (8 repetitions per set)

• Dumbbell Kickback – Perform 3 sets of 8 repetitions per set.

• Perform 3 sets of Inclined Dumbbell Flyes, with 12 repetitions in each set.

• Vigorous Cardiovascular Exercise – 20 minutes

Day 3

• Moderate-intensity cardiovascular exercise – Duration of 30 to 45 minutes.

Day 4

• Sumo Deadlift: Perform 3 sets, with 8 repetitions per set.

• Perform 20 repetitions of kettlebell swings, dividing them into multiple sets.

• Three sets of chest supported rows with eight repetitions per set.

• Preacher Curl – Perform 3 sets of 8 repetitions per set.

• Perform three sets of reverse grip pull-down, with each set comprising of twelve repetitions.

• Vigorous cardiovascular exercise – 20 minutes

Day 5

• Three sets of military press, with eight repetitions per set.

• Medicine Ball Overthrow – Perform 20 repetitions, dividing them into several sets.

• Cable Lateral Raise – Three sets comprising eight repetitions per set.

• Three sets of rear delt raises with eight repetitions each will be performed. • The exercise routine will include three sets of rear delt raises, with eight repetitions in each set. • The prescribed workout plan involves three sets comprising of eight reps each for the rear delt raises.

• Barbell Roll-Out– Perform 3 sets with 12 repetitions per set.

- Perform the Dead Bug exercise for a total of 3 sets, with each set consisting of 12 repetitions.

• Cardiovascular Exercise with High Intensity - duration of 20 minutes

Days 6 and 7 will be designated for relaxation and recuperation.
During the designated time period of Block 3, which spans over Weeks 9 to 12,

With the objective of augmenting the resistance applied to principal movements, modifications will be made to both the primary and ancillary exercises. Exert rigorous effort, as the level of intensity held is of utmost importance.

Day 1

• X-Band Walk – Perform 3 sets consisting of 8 repetitions in each direction.

• Execute 20 repetitions of Box Jumps, distributing them across multiple sets.

• Leg Extensions – Perform 3 sets, with 8 repetitions per set.

• Seated Single-Leg Curl – 3 sets (8 reps per set)

• Back Squat – Perform 3 sets with 12 repetitions per set.

• Three sets of standing calf raises, with 12 repetitions per set.

• Twenty minutes of high-intensity cardiovascular exercise

Day 2

• Three sets of barbell bench press, with each set consisting of eight repetitions.

- Medicine Ball Pass - Perform 20 repetitions, divided into multiple sets.

- Cable Cross-Over – Perform 3 sets consisting of 8 repetitions per set.

- Perform three sets of overhead dumbbell tricep exercises, with eight repetitions per set.

- Bench Dip - Perform 3 sets consisting of 12 repetitions per set.

- Vigorous Cardiovascular Activity – 20 minutes

Day 3

- Duration of low-intensity cardiovascular exercise: 30 to 45 minutes

Day 4

• The deadlift exercise should be completed in three sets, with each set consisting of eight repetitions.

• Perform 20 repetitions of kettlebell swings, partitioned into several sets.

• Perform three sets of Pull-Ups, with eight repetitions per set.

• Execute three sets comprising eight repetitions per set of the exercise titled Alternating Dumbbell Curl.

• Cable Row – Perform 3 sets consisting of 12 repetitions per set.

• 20 minutes of high-intensity cardiovascular exercise

Day 5

• Engage in the push press exercise for a total of 5 sets, with each set consisting of 5 repetitions.

• Perform a total of 20 repetitions of the Medicine Ball Overthrow exercise, dividing it into multiple sets.

• Three sets of barbell roll-out, with eight repetitions per set.

• Execute three sets of alternating dumbbell curls, with eight repetitions per set.

• The last row of the arrangement - 3 sets (with 12 repetitions per set)

• Vigorous Cardiovascular Exercise – 20 minutes

Incorporating Days 6 and 7 into the schedule for rest and recuperation.

If one is inclined to design their own weight training program, it is advisable to incorporate certain components, such as supplementary exercises, multi-joint exercises, and cardiovascular routines that align with one's objectives. Adhere to your established regimen and exert your utmost effort. Exercise patience and unwavering perseverance, and you will witness the fruits of your labor.

Chapter Three: Expert Techniques and Strategies

These strategies will assist you in executing programs to meet your specific objectives. As your objectives evolve, such as transitioning from muscle gain to fat reduction, it becomes necessary to adapt certain methodologies accordingly.

Consume a substantial morning meal

Bodybuilding diets consistently advocate for a substantial breakfast that is rich in protein and complex carbohydrates. Whether your goal is to reduce body fat or increase muscle mass, consuming a substantial breakfast initiates your metabolism, supplying you with the necessary calories and nutrients to initiate and sustain your daily activities.

Consume multiple meals throughout the day.

It is advisable for individuals engaged in bodybuilding to consume a maximum number of meals, aiming to have at least five meals per day during rest days and a total of seven meals on workout days. Consuming multiple meals serves numerous purposes. It ensures the continuous supply of essential micro- and macronutrients to support the process of muscle development.

Maintaining a consistent intake of calories aids in sustaining an elevated metabolic rate, increasing the likelihood of utilizing energy rather than storing it as body fat.

Include a small pre-exercise meal.

The previous convention was to engage in training sessions while refraining from consuming any food. Research indicates that the consumption of a modest meal, ideally consisting of approximately 20 grams of protein in the form of a shake, such as whey, along with roughly 20-40 grams of carbohydrates with a slow digestion rate, such as fruit, immediately prior to exercising (within a timeframe of 15 to 30 minutes), can effectively enhance energy levels during the workout and contribute to improved recovery and muscular development after exercising.

Minimize the intake of carbohydrates during subsequent meals.

In a similar vein, I suggest consuming the majority of your carbohydrates earlier in the day and during your exercise routine, and it is also advisable to gradually reduce carbohydrate intake as the day advances. Subsequently, particularly subsequent to your meals following physical exertion, there is diminished necessity for calories that contribute to energy production, thereby resulting in their effortless accumulation as adipose tissue.

Refrain from consuming unhealthy food options such as junk foods and processed foods.

The allurements are pervasive – carbonated beverages, quick-service meals, and snack items. You are advised to refrain from consuming these evidently high-sugar and high-fat adversaries (even while experiencing hunger). Unproductive caloric content pervades the American culinary landscape, particularly in social gatherings, yet accomplished bodybuilders possess the skill to engage in conversations without indulging in unwarranted consumption. Consumption of refined grain products, such as donuts and white bread, can have a deleterious impact on one's physical well-being. Even the beverage commonly known as lemonade may contain a higher sugar content than actual lemon. Processed cold cuts, due to their inclusion of nitrates and preservatives, deviate significantly from authentic lean meat. Learn the difference.

Utilize designated rest days for the purpose of nourishment, incorporating them as nutrition-focused days.

Frequently, bodybuilders perceive a rest day as a period of time detached from their bodybuilding endeavors. There is nothing to the contrary. One does not experience growth during the training, but rather it is during the recovery phase from training that growth occurs. The human body possesses the ability to restore itself efficiently when it is not exposed to the strain of heavy weights. A non-training day presents an optimal occasion for you to consume bodybuilding foods, although it is important to exercise caution and attentiveness in managing your diet. Do not consume an excess amount of calories beyond your necessary intake. By emphasizing the consumption of lean protein and high-quality complex carbohydrates, you can significantly enhance your ability to effectively develop muscle mass.

Plan Ahead

Occasionally, work commitments, academic timetables, or travel arrangements may disrupt one's dietary routine. Prevent regression in nutritional habits through proactive planning. Creating meals in advance, utilizing Tupperware containers, and carrying meal-replacement powders or protein bars with you are a few straightforward strategies to ensure the fulfillment of your nutritional needs regardless of the demands presented by your circumstances. Certain seasoned bodybuilders prepare a week's worth of meals in a single evening, ensuring their readiness to perform efficiently when schedules become constrained.

Freezers, preserved food items, microwave ovens, plastic storage containers, and prepackaged nutritional supplements are all resources that enable individuals to maintain a ready supply of substantial meals for their busy lifestyles.

Additional Recommendations and Strategies for Slender Individuals to Efficiently Gain Muscle Mass Speedily

Individuals with a slender physique often encounter significant challenges in their efforts to build muscle mass. Regardless of their efforts, they consistently encounter difficulties in acquiring weight and muscle mass.

Additionally, it is observed that they do not typically exhibit a propensity for weight gain. However, it is truly vexing to witness individuals who do not exert the same level of effort in their fitness routines obtain larger muscle mass and a more formidable physique.

What actions can be taken with regard to this situation?

Allow me to present you with additional recommendations that you should consider incorporating into your exercise regimen, with the aim of efficiently enhancing muscle growth and transforming them into formidable muscular strength.

Excessive reliance on training to failure may impede your growth.

Several individuals propose that training to failure is necessary to achieve optimal muscle growth. I hold a contrasting viewpoint on this matter, and opine that it would be advantageous for a hardgainer to refrain from engaging in this particular form of training in order to truly observe significant outcomes.

Consider this... if I were to propose that you engage in a full-out sprint around a 400-meter track, you would likely find yourself struggling for breath and unable to sustain the initial pace, reaching only halfway. In the gym as well, an excessive workload at an early stage will impede the optimization of your entire exercise routine.

Please do not misunderstand me, it is advisable not to restrain yourself during your workouts... nevertheless, refrain from performing an excessive number of repetitions until your body reaches a point where it is no longer able to continue.

Develop Muscular Strength During Rest

The importance of adequately allocating time for sleep is frequently disregarded in almost all exercise regimens. Contemporary society appears to encourage individuals to maximize their time utilization, even at the expense of sacrificing their sleep. Insufficient sleep will unquestionably impede your muscle development.

Why? An increase in endogenous levels of anabolic growth hormones occurs during periods of sleep, especially during deep sleep. Therefore, obtaining a sufficient duration of sleep, ideally around 8 hours, can be highly beneficial for individuals aiming to expedite muscle growth.

The absence of sufficient sleep not only prevents the body from receiving the advantages of the anabolic growth hormone but also compels a more unfavorable condition. Elevated levels of catabolic hormones, such as Cortisol, are observed when there is insufficient sleep, which has the counterproductive effect of diminishing anabolic hormones. In other words, these hormones deplete muscle mass. If one consistently obtains only four or five hours of sleep per night, they may potentially diminish their muscle size instead of enhancing it. Incorporate sufficient time for sleep and rest within your hardgainer workout regimen.

Engaging in resistance training exercises with low repetitions and heavy weights contributes to muscle development.

Do not succumb to the deceptive belief of pursuing 'high sets, high reps'. High repetitions are highly efficacious for enhancing toning, achieving definition, and improving muscular endurance. However, they are unequivocally unfavorable for individuals aiming to augment their muscle mass.

Adhering to a low repetition scheme with heavy weights, executed with notable intensity, is recommended. A muscle will only develop if it is compelled to do so. If one possesses the capability to perform a substantial quantity of repetitions, it indicates that their muscle has adapted to the resistance and is prepared to handle an increased workload.

All whole-body exercises are superior to isolation exercises.

Adhere to the fundamental compound exercises including squats, deadlifts, bicep curls, bench press, bent over rows, woodchoppers, and so forth. These exercises are widely recognized and favored by all bodybuilders. Why do you believe that individuals who achieve the distinction of winning the Mr. Universe titles continue to engage in these physical routines? It is because they diligently engage in physical exertion, fostering the development of remarkable muscularity and fortitude unparalleled by any other endeavors.

Muscle Development - Strategies for Achieving Substantial Muscle Growth for Individuals with Difficulty Gaining Mass

Individuals with difficulty gaining muscle mass frequently, if not invariably, belong to the somatotype classification known as ectomorph. Individuals belonging to this classification typically possess a slender physique and exhibit a petite structure.

They frequently struggle with weight gain, and are capable of consuming nearly anything without experiencing any increase in body mass. It can be challenging for these individuals to attain significant muscle growth due to the apparent acceleration of their metabolism with increased food consumption. Nonetheless, it is not an insurmountable feat to increase muscle mass, even though one may not achieve significant size; nevertheless, it is still possible to cultivate a remarkable physique.

The most crucial factor for hard gainers who aim to increase their muscle mass is undeniably their dietary intake. It is imperative that you partake in the consumption of food, and do so in significant quantities. Right when one believes they have consumed enough, they find themselves needing to partake in another serving. It is necessary for you to determine your daily caloric requirements and subsequently increase your intake by an additional 1000-1500 calories. If an individual requires 2500 calories per day to sustain their current weight, it is advisable to consume approximately 3500-4000 calories on a daily basis. The recommended dietary components consist of quality complex carbohydrates and protein. In the event that you are unable to achieve this through the consumption of solid food, you have the option to purchase weight gain supplementation and protein powder. However, the majority of your daily nutrition must be derived from solid wholesome foods.

Hard gainers, also known as ectomorphs, should adhere to compound exercises such as the bench press, military press, squats, deadlifts, and skull crushers when engaging in weightlifting. These exercises prioritize multiple muscle groups simultaneously, thereby promoting enhanced muscular growth. It is equally important to adhere to the range of 6-8 repetitions, typically with approximately 3-4 sets. Periodically, in order to diversify the strain on your muscles, you may incorporate power sets into your exercise regimen, wherein you adhere to performing 6-8 repetitions for 2-3 sets.

Rest is crucial because individuals with ectomorphic physiques experience rapid muscle fatigue and require more time for recovery compared to individuals with other body types. Hard gainers have been known to invest

Spending extensive periods of time at the gym often yields limited or negligible outcomes, and in certain instances, individuals may experience a decline in muscle mass and physical power. As an individual with difficulty in building muscle mass, I have come to understand that a minimalist approach produces superior results when engaging in weightlifting activities. It is advisable that you limit your workout sessions to focusing on 1-2 specific body parts, while ensuring that you allow for a period of 1-2 days of rest between each session. Cardiovascular exercise should only be incorporated into one's routine 2-3 times per week, with each session lasting no more than approximately 30 minutes; since it is not advisable to expend any additional calories.

Enhancement should encompass the incorporation of a multivitamin, protein powder, and an oil rich in omega 3-6 fatty acids. These products will aid in restoring your body's vitamin and mineral levels, which may be depleted during your exercise sessions. This will facilitate expedited muscle recovery as well.

Attaining weight for individuals with a naturally slender physique is inherently challenging and necessitates considerable dedication and effort. Nevertheless, if you maintain consistency in your nutritional habits, weightlifting sessions, and resting periods, you will undoubtedly observe significant progress in a short period of time.

Enhancing Lower Body Muscle Growth: The Definitive Regimen

When closely scrutinizing matters of significance, one often discovers that there exists a depth beyond initial perceptions. Consider this lower-body metabolic exercise routine as an illustrative example. Upon initial inspection, it may appear quite rudimentary. However, I strongly encourage you to attempt it precisely as I have recommended. Exhibit a rigorous adherence to structure and punctuality, and you will expeditiously realize that success lies not in the actions undertaken, but rather in the meticulous execution thereof.

The skeletal system of the human body possesses blood vessels that bear a striking resemblance to the intricate network of root systems found in trees. At the outset, the primary root exhibits significant thickness, which subsequently bifurcates into more delicate subsidiary roots that extend extensively in quest of nourishment. The arterial system of the human body exhibits significant resemblance to arteries serving as the primary conduits through which oxygenated blood is supplied to the muscles. Subsequently, these arteries give rise to an intricate network of capillaries spanning the entirety of the muscular tissue. During a state of rest, blood circulates through these arteries; however, it is noteworthy that merely 30% of these arterial vessels are replenished with fresh blood with each cardiac contraction. The remaining 70% comprises blood that is stagnant in circulation but rich in oxygen, awaiting movement. Please take a moment to consider the following, as it involves a certain level of depth. If you do not immediately grasp the concept, I urge you to reread it.

In customary practice, the comprehensive utilization of muscles is seldom achieved during exercise, with approximately 30% of muscle fibers being primarily responsible for the exertion. Upon the conclusion of the exercise regimen, one experiences a sense of having exerted maximum effort; nonetheless, aside from some minor discomfort, there is minimal enhancement in endurance, strength, or hypertrophy subsequently. The absence of substantial progress leads to the onset of frustration, prompting individuals to resort to adding more resistance. However, besides increasing the risk of injury, this strategy yields minimal results and instead impairs the same 30% of muscle fibers. Consequently, the muscle becomes overtrained and instinctively attempts to recover in a slightly contracted and inflexible condition. This phenomenon gradually evolves into the adhesion occurring among adjacent muscles, which subsequently leads to eventual injury.

Provided that you comprehend all of the aforementioned, I shall now proceed to outline the exercise regimen for you to adhere to. However, I advise you to remain attentive for an upcoming video that will be included in the question and answer segment, which will expound upon this matter with greater elaboration.

The exercise routine comprises of three exercises targeting the Quadriceps, Hamstrings, and Calves. These exercises are designed as a warm-up and pre-fatigue method, gradually increasing blood flow to the muscles in the lower body. This prepares the muscles for the final exercise, which will subject them to complete failure through overload. The pace for the elongation of the muscle is two seconds, with one second at both the peak and the nadir of the motion, and a final one second for the contraction of the muscle.

Perform 12 repetitions, complete 3 sets, and allow a 60-second interval between sets before proceeding to the subsequent exercise.

Exercise 1 is Leg Extension, exercise 2 corresponds to Lying Leg Curl, and exercise 3 pertains to Donkey Calf Raises.

Upon completion of the previous set, proceed to perform three sets of barbell squats consisting of 12 repetitions each.

Gradually increase the weight for each set, while allowing one minute of rest between sets.

Exercise 4a involves performing barbell squats, with a total workout duration of 23 minutes.

If you lack a secure method for performing Barbell Squats and desire to utilize Dumbbells instead, the following course of action may be pursued. Choose a set of dumbbells equivalent to 85% of the weight used for the Barbell Squat, while ensuring that the tempo consists of a 2-second descent and a swift ascent. Perform 12 repetitions, followed by a 10-second rest period, repeat the process for another 12 repetitions, rest for 10 seconds again, and conclude with a final set of 12 repetitions.

Exercise 4b stands as a viable substitute for Barbell Squats. Dumbbell Squats. Place a 2cm block beneath your heels or utilize a 1.25kg weight plate. This task is expected to be completed within a time frame of approximately 2 minutes. Be sure to execute a controlled descent, maintaining a lowered position for a duration of two seconds, and subsequently initiate a rapid ascension without pausing at the extremes of the movement. Perform this exercise a total of twelve times, followed by a ten-second interval of rest, while maintaining an upright standing position and grasping the dumbbells. After a brief interval of 10 seconds, proceed to perform an additional set of 12 repetitions. Take another 10-second break followed by the completion of your final set, consisting of 12 repetitions.

Hence, the overall duration of the workout when substituting exercise 4b for exercise 4a amounts to 20 minutes.

Beginning Bodybuilding

Bodybuilding entails engaging in progressive resistance exercise techniques to cultivate and enhance muscular development. An individual involved in this form of pursuit is referred to as a bodybuilder. Bodybuilding is an athletic pursuit that necessitates substantial discipline from the practitioner. Through exerting control, you are able to maintain consistency by adhering to a structured exercise regimen. Dedicated bodybuilders exhibit unwavering discipline by persevering through their workouts regardless of external conditions, including inclement weather or personal fatigue. They ensure that they are mindful of their dietary choices. If one aspires to pursue a career in professional bodybuilding, it is imperative to exhibit unwavering focus and engage in rigorous and intensive training.

How to start bodybuilding

If you possess a sincere desire to improve your physical condition but find yourself uncertain of the appropriate initial steps, the following recommendations may prove beneficial, particularly for individuals who are new to the realm of bodybuilding. These are recommendations that you can integrate into your daily regimen. One may inquire, delve further into literature, conduct extensive research, and experiment with various methodologies. Prior to commencing, obtain a medical clearance from a qualified physician.

1. Engage in a quest to find a fitness facility

Identify a suitable location wherein the majority of your bodybuilding endeavors and fitness regimens will take place. Opt for a gym facility that upholds cleanliness standards and is equipped with state-of-the-art exercise apparatus. Additionally, it is crucial to ascertain the availability of knowledgeable personnel and trainers. In order to prevent the use of excuses for not attending the gym, it would be wise to locate a facility that is conveniently located either in close proximity to your residence or within reasonable distance of your workplace.

2. Set realistic goals

Establish objectives that can be realistically achieved within a defined time frame. It is important to ensure that the goals you set are achievable, as unrealistic ones may result in disappointment upon their eventual realization. Start small. Establish attainable objectives at a comfortable speed.

One of the primary objectives you desire to accomplish is the enhancement of both muscular strength and mass within your physique. Upon honing your muscular strength, you may commence the process of refining their appearance.

When devising strategies to achieve your objectives, adopt a proper mental framework. Exercising patience and maintaining a steadfast commitment will assist you in overcoming challenges.

3. Please give careful consideration to your physical well-being.

Pay heed to the messages conveyed by your physical being. If you are not sufficiently capable - not due to idleness, but rather due to feelings of physical weakness or nausea, abstain from your workout and return to the gym once you have made a significant improvement.

Exerting minimal effort during a workout while experiencing physical discomfort yields no productive results.

4. Acquire a dependable training companion.

Having a trustworthy training companion proves immensely beneficial in the pursuit of muscle gain or professional bodybuilding. Your partner can play a significant role in aiding you in the attainment of your bodybuilding objectives. By engaging in a fitness partnership, a dynamic of healthy competition is fostered, leading to accelerated progress for both individuals involved.

5. Stretching

Prior to commencing the exercise routine, it is advisable to engage in muscle stretching and warming up activities to enhance blood circulation. Commence your workout routine by engaging in low-intensity cardiovascular exercises and performing targeted stretches for the muscles that you intend to focus on during your training session.

6. Proper Breathing

One technique employed in the realm of bodybuilding and weightlifting entails the practice of appropriate respiration, as it facilitates the provision of oxygen to the muscular system, thereby playing a vital role in fostering their growth and facilitating their controlled contraction.

The recommended action is to expel breath while lifting and inhale while lowering the weight.

7. Bodybuilding for Beginners

Novice individuals will require proper guidance regarding the initiation of bodybuilding activities.

8. Train in cycles

If you are a newcomer, you may be contemplating the frequency at which each muscle group should be trained. It is customary to observe a period of 48 hours before engaging in the training of a muscle group for a second time. By employing this approach, you will facilitate the creation of training cycles. Additionally, please remember to allocate a day for recuperation to allow your body to rejuvenate.

9. Proper diet

One may engage in weightlifting to their desired extent, but it is imperative to concurrently adhere to a suitable dietary regimen. Failure to do so will result in the failure to achieve desired outcomes. It is imperative to uphold a well-balanced dietary regime by ensuring the appropriate intake of calories from varying food categories, specifically fats, protein, and carbohydrates. Vitamins and minerals hold significant importance as well.

The dietary needs of individuals will vary based on their weight and fitness objectives. In general, it is advisable to consume smaller portions and eat with greater frequency as opposed to consuming a single large meal. Ensure adequate hydration by consuming a generous amount of water.

10. Do sets and reps of different exercises

It is necessary to perform varying sets and repetitions of distinct exercises. The number of repetitions performed consecutively will denote the quantity of times an exercise is executed in a sequence, whereas a set pertains to the consecutive block of repetitions for a specific exercise.

As an illustration, should you choose to engage in three sets of 15 repetitions of push-ups, you would be required to consecutively perform three clusters of 15 push-ups each.

11. Combine aerobics and cardio

After acquiring proficiency in bodybuilding and attaining a fundamental understanding of weightlifting techniques, incorporate 2 to 3 cardiovascular training sessions per week into your routine. This will assist in fat burning, promote cardiovascular health, and alleviate stress.

12. Supplements

Enhance your journey towards achieving professional bodybuilding status by incorporating protein powders into your regimen. This is strongly recommended for novice individuals aiming to achieve lean muscle mass. Protein shakes serve as a convenient option for consumption during interim periods between meals.

13. Rest and relaxation

Following an extensive workout session, it is essential for your body to have a period of rest. Ensure that you obtain sufficient rest during the night and refrain from excessive physical exertion during exercise and other activities. During the rest period, your muscles undergo the process of nutrient absorption from protein intake to facilitate their growth and development.

14. Training log

Maintain diligent records of your progression in bodybuilding and consistently document your workouts in a structured training log. Please transcribe the exercise regimen, including the series and repetitions performed during the workout. This can provide you with a future focus and a means of monitoring your advancement.

17. Essential Information Regarding Muscle Building

Are you seeking to enhance muscular strength and size? There are numerous strategies available to enhance your muscle-building outcomes and optimize workout efficiency. If your aim is to increase both size and strength, this article can provide valuable guidance to help you achieve your objectives. Cease the inefficient use of time within the gym and avail yourself of these efficacious recommendations.

Direct your attention towards critical exercises like the deadlift, squat, and bench press. These exercises are fundamental for bodybuilders. They have the potential to enhance physical strength, foster endurance, and optimize the efficacy of subsequent exercise sessions. It is advisable to regularly incorporate them into your daily activities.

I would recommend making an effort to alter your established regimen. Engaging in the same exercise regimen repeatedly can lead to monotony, thereby impeding your motivation to engage in physical activity. Please ensure to consistently maintain your exercise regimen by utilizing various gym equipment or availing yourself of diverse exercise classes. By ensuring variety and novelty in your exercise regimen, you can cultivate sustained engagement and dedication to your muscle-building endeavors.

Compound exercises hold significant importance in the process of muscle development. These exercises engage multiple muscle groups simultaneously during the lifting motion. As an example, the exercise of bench pressing serves to facilitate the development of various muscle groups including the shoulders, chest, and triceps.

When engaging in physical exercise, it is crucial to engage various muscle groups during training sessions, such as combining pectoral exercises with dorsal exercises, or incorporating hamstring exercises along with quadriceps exercises. This protocol facilitates muscle relaxation during the activation of its counteracting counterpart. Consequently, by constraining the duration of your gym sessions, you can effectively enhance the intensity of your workouts.

Plyometric exercises provide an optimal method for muscular development. These types of exercises will aid in the improvement of your fast twitch muscles, thereby promoting more extensive muscle growth. Plyometrics bear resemblance to ballistic exercises in that they necessitate the presence of acceleration. For instance, in the case of engaging in plyometric push-ups, the act entails lifting your hands off the ground, leading to the upward propulsion of your body.

It is permissible to employ minor modifications in technique while engaging in weightlifting endeavors. Utilizing the mechanical advantage of your body weight to extract additional repetitions is a straightforward method to enhance the outcomes of your workout regime. Please exercise caution to avoid engaging in cheating frequently. Ensure that you maintain a controlled speed while performing repetitions. Please refrain from compromising your posture/technique.

The three fundamental exercises for increasing muscle mass are the squat, the bench press, and the deadlift, often referred to as the sacred triad. Through the engagement in these exercises, one will swiftly develop muscular strength and achieve a desirable level of physical fitness. You have the option to incorporate additional exercises into your fitness routine, however, those three exercises should constitute the fundamental basis of it.

It is not advisable to perform all exercises with heavier weights. Excessive weight placed on your joints during neck exercises, dips, and split squats can potentially result in severe injury to oneself. Alternatively, employ higher resistance loads predominantly for workouts involving rows, presses, deadlifts, and squats.

Apply cognitive abilities while performing squats. Place the barbell on your upper back, aligning it with the midpoint of your trapezius muscles. By engaging in this action, you impose additional strain on the muscles situated in the lower extremities, specifically encompassing the quadriceps, glutes, and hip region. Utilizing these muscles will enable you to increase your lifting capacity.

Ensure that you have a clear understanding of the capabilities and limitations of your physique. This will assist you in acquiring a comprehensive comprehension of your objectives and your starting position. Ensure that you take into account parameters such as body weight, body fat percentage, and any underlying health considerations when undertaking a personal assessment.

This article exemplifies that there are various methodologies one can adopt to build muscle, and it is likely that some approaches will yield better results for individuals than others. By implementing these recommendations, you can expedite the development of lean muscle mass. Optimize the benefits of your muscle building workouts by utilizing this valuable information.

18. Strategies for Enhancing Muscle Development

Anyone can build muscle. It is possible that you may not have considered this, yet the strategies that have proven effective for others can also be beneficial for you. It is essential to acquire the appropriate methodologies and employ them to benefit oneself. This article will elucidate several empirically validated approaches for acquiring muscular mass.

It is imperative to integrate an ample quantity of vegetables into your dietary intake. Though diets that prioritize muscle growth typically emphasize the consumption of carbohydrates and protein, they often neglect the importance of incorporating vegetables into one's meal plan. Vegetables possess vital nutrients that are not found in other carbohydrate and protein-rich foods. They can also serve as excellent sources of dietary fiber. Dietary fiber enables the body to enhance its utilization of ingested protein.

Direct your attention towards the dead lift, the bench press, and the squat. Each of these exercises is believed to serve as the foundation for effective bodybuilding regimens, a statement that holds true. Seasoned bodybuilders are aware that not only do they contribute to fundamental conditioning, but they also enhance muscular strength and facilitate hypertrophy. Regardless of the variations you incorporate into your routine, it is essential to consistently engage in these fundamental exercises.

Introduce periodic alterations to your exercise regimen on a weekly basis. After a period of extended exercise, it is possible to experience a sense of monotony towards your current fitness regimen. This can result in the depletion of your motivation and ultimately lead to complete cessation of your fitness regime. Variate your exercise routine in every workout session to ensure engagement of distinct muscle groups each time. By modifying your exercise regimens, you maintain their novelty and ensure sustained involvement.

If your intention is to prepare for a marathon or any other athletic competition, abstain from attempting to concurrently enhance muscular development. Engaging in cardiovascular exercise can be beneficial for maintaining fitness, but an excessive amount of it may impede progress in developing muscle mass. When endeavoring to enhance your muscle mass, prioritize strength-focused exercises while slightly reducing the emphasis on conditioning.

Do not overlook the importance of carbohydrates in your muscle-building endeavors. Carbohydrates provide the necessary energy to support daily physical exercise requirements. In the event that your training regimen is comprehensive, it may be necessary to augment your daily intake of carbohydrates to a range of 2-3 grams per pound of body weight.

Compound exercises are an excellent means of efficiently engaging in comprehensive strength training within a limited time frame. These exercises have been specifically formulated to engage various muscle groups through integrated movements. An exemplary instance of a compound exercise is the execution of a shoulder press while in a squat stance, effectively engaging both the lower body and the shoulder muscles concurrently.

Ensuring proper hydration of your body constitutes a crucial element of a well-rounded muscle-development regimen. To mitigate the risk of personal harm, it is imperative to maintain adequate levels of hydration. Optimal hydration additionally constitutes a vital aspect in the sustenance and advancement of muscle mass, rendering it a crucial determinant for multiple purposes.

It is permissible to employ certain strategies to expedite the process of weightlifting. If you wish to maximize the effectiveness of your exercise routine by adding a few additional repetitions, it is advised to refrain from exerting excessive strain on your entire physique. However, it is crucial to ensure that cheating is kept at a minimum. Please ensure that the pace of your repetitions remains steady. Ensure that your form remains uncompromised. Developing a timetable for your fitness regime can enable you to optimize your ability to build muscle and minimize the risk of injury. For novice individuals, it is advised to partake in challenging exercise routines no more frequently than twice per week. As for more experienced individuals, the option to incorporate an additional day into their workout schedule is available.

If one demonstrates unwavering commitment, muscle development can be attained. Adhere to the recommendations delineated in this article to facilitate the process. You are poised for success in achieving the desired physique by effectively incorporating accurate information into your bodybuilding regimen.

Training Intensity

Very well, let's add some excitement to the situation. Up to this point, we have covered the concepts of volume and frequency and populated our agenda with several practical exercises. Nevertheless, if these three factors were the sole determinants in muscle development, it would follow that individuals engaging in consistent dumbbell exercises would inevitably possess significantly augmented arm muscles. So, why don't they?

They fail to do so because several crucial elements are yet to be included, with training intensity being one of them. To stimulate hypertrophy, it is imperative that exercises are performed with sufficient intensity. Alternatively, one could potentially develop their biceps by engaging in the activity of air curls on a regular basis, which could be deemed as a favorable outcome. You may find it amusing, but there are indeed female influencers who actively endorse arm workouts focused on weight reduction and muscle building, among other similar concepts...

Training intensity refers to the magnitude of weight employed during sets relative to an individual's one repetition maximum. Do not misconstrue it as relative intensity or relative effort, which pertains to the perceived level of difficulty during your workout set—this will be discussed in detail subsequently.

Intensity is commonly expressed as a percentage and is marginally more predominant in the realm of strength training in comparison to bodybuilding communities. Individuals in the field of bodybuilding are likely to possess a deeper understanding of incorporating repetition ranges into their training regime; nonetheless, it should be emphasized that these two concepts essentially convey an identical meaning.

As an illustration, let us consider a scenario where your present maximum weight that you can lift during a bench press is 100 kg. Should you commence your set with a load of 80 kg, it would be deemed that you are engaging in training with an intensity level of 80%. Subsequently, it becomes inconsequential whether you perform a single repetition or continue until muscle failure, as the intensity of this set remained at 80%.

"If you harbor an inclination, here are the prevailing proportions (articulated in repetitions):

The maximal weight that can be lifted for one repetition, representing the complete exertion of strength.

Based on the given data, the 2 rep maximum weight capacity reaches 95%.

According to data, a 90% 4-repetition maximum (4RM) was achieved.

Based on the maximum number of repetitions, the weight can be lifted at an approximate rate of 85%, assuming the individual can perform 6 repetitions.

Eighty percent of the maximum weight that can be lifted for a total of eight repetitions.

A 75% intensity level corresponding to a maximum weight of 10 repetitions.

Seventy percent of the 12 repetition maximum.

A rep max of 16 corresponds to 65%

Sixty percent of the twenty repetition maximum

A reduction of 50% in the maximum repetition weight.

Nowadays, it is widely recognized even by novice individuals that they must subject themselves to a sufficient level of intensity during training in order to stimulate muscle growth. Therefore, the sole inquiries that remain are:

What is heavy enough?

What is too heavy?

What is too light?

Fortuitously, there has been extensive research conducted on rep ranges and training intensity pertaining to hypertrophy, yielding commendable guidelines. According to research, levels of intensity between approximately 50% and 85% of one's maximum weight capacity are deemed to be optimal for pure hypertrophy.

Based on scientific evidence, it has been observed that a range of five to 30 repetitions, while factoring in the presence of reserve repetitions, can contribute to an approximately equal muscle-building effect.

Therefore, engaging in excessive physical exertion at rep ranges below five is likely to be excessively burdensome, resulting in suboptimal outcomes in terms of muscle development. Sets of this magnitude are more apt for focusing on building strength and have the potential to hinder your overall workload capacity if you exceed your limits or strain your joints excessively. A comprehensive analysis demonstrated that individuals must engage in a regimen consisting of seven demanding sets of three repetitions to achieve an equivalent level of hypertrophy as that attained through three challenging sets of ten repetitions.

In contrast, should you opt for a lighter load, you would primarily target your muscular endurance and risk neglecting the activation of your fast twitch fibers, which are essential for substantial growth. Have you ever observed a cyclist participating in the Tour de France, known for their well-developed lower extremities? Now you know why.

Nevertheless, from my perspective, the scientific guidelines suggesting a range of 30 (or potentially 40) repetitions per set are unduly extravagant. These sets with high repetitions will require approximately two minutes or longer to finish, thereby rendering them relatively inefficient in terms of time utilization, given that the majority of those repetitions are solely aimed at achieving the desired outcome. Nevertheless, the primary concern lies in the fact that, eventually, the severe discomfort and muscular fatigue become so excessive that there is a potential likelihood of terminating your sets prematurely, well before reaching the point of muscle failure. And as you are about to discover in the subsequent chapter, that is not recommended if your intention is to achieve significant benefits.

Regarding the optimal range for hypertrophy, I would suggest that a rep range of anywhere from 5 to 20 repetitions per set is highly effective.

Novice individuals may find it advantageous to initially prioritize a middle range approach, focusing on performing heavier sets in the range of 8–12 repetitions. When appropriately managed in terms of relative effort (i.e., ensuring that intensity is not pushed to the point of failure), this approach substantially reduces the likelihood of sustaining injuries. Additionally, it affords you the opportunity to acquire a safer approach in mastering the more intricate barbell exercises, without sacrificing their effectiveness. For less demanding tasks, you might consider operating within the scope of the 12–15 range at approximately 65% effort, as well as the 15–20 range at around 60% exertion level, which is what I personally adopt. Please be aware that this is a purely subjective decision without any specific reason or logic behind it. A recommended range for repetitions serves the purpose of confining your sets within a specific and narrower range of repetitions, which is crucial for the purposes of progression (but further elaboration on this matter will be provided subsequently).

Furthermore, through incorporating a well-balanced combination of both intense and moderate exercises into your training regimen, you can effectively target your muscles from multiple angles:

The higher-intensity exercise is highly effective in engaging all muscle fibers, particularly the fast-twitch type-II fibers that are more responsive to growth stimulus, while also generating substantial muscular tension.

The lower-intensity exercise effectively targets intermediate and slow twitch muscle fibers and induces muscular hypertrophy by generating metabolic stress.

When embarking upon the process of developing a program, I would recommend commencing with approximately 66% to 75% of the complete number of sets allocated for each major muscle group, within the higher to moderate intensity thresholds (specifically, within the range of 6 to 10 repetitions and 8 to 12 repetitions). For the remaining options, it is advisable to choose lighter variations within the ranges of 12–15, 15-20, and so forth. I frequently discover it more advantageous to adhere to elevated repetition ranges when exercising smaller muscle groups. Exercises such as calf raises or crunches performed in sets of six may not be sufficient for the majority of individuals.

However, it should be noted that rep ranges are subjective and can vary based on individual preferences and level of expertise. It is possible to observe that certain muscle groups exhibit a remarkable response to higher intensities of exercise, while displaying less or no response to lower intensities - or vice versa. It could potentially be specific to a particular form of physical activity. Certain exercises are more appropriate for higher levels of intensity, while others are more suited for lower levels of intensity. For instance, consistently performing deadlifts in sets of 20 or engaging in sets of five side-lateral raises may not offer the most optimal results. Please kindly consider revisiting the Exercise chapter of this book for further guidance on recommendations pertaining to each exercise. Generally speaking, if one utilizes a barbell, they are able to engage in substantial resistance training. If one engages in exercises utilizing dumbbells or cables, it may be advisable to opt for lighter weights.

As an illustration, when engaging in bench presses within the 6-10 repetition range, a notable increase in muscle pump and a distinct sensation of chest muscle activation are experienced. However, executing 15 repetitions per set yields ineffective results for me. In contrast, squats exhibit a dissimilar effect: engaging in low repetitions depletes my energy levels on a systemic scale, although my quadriceps muscles appear to be relatively unaffected. However, are you referring to performing sets consisting of 10 repetitions? Remarkably, these exercises exert an incredibly intense strain on my quadriceps muscles.

An additional principle to consider would involve commencing your fitness routines with higher levels of exertion and focal compound movements, and concluding with decreased levels of effort and isolated movements. Compound exercises combined with high intensities provide substantial efficiency and should not be compromised by pre-exhausting the intended muscles (typically, at the very least). Additionally, these fundamental exercises often entail a higher level of technical proficiency, and it is imperative that your form remains intact even when fatigued.

After becoming proficient in exercises targeting major muscle groups within the 8–12 repetition range, such as deadlifts, squats, bench presses, and similar exercises, and gaining confidence in performing them, consider progressing to more demanding intensities in your subsequent mesocycle, where the repetition range would be around 6–10 (~75% of maximum) instead.

On occasion, when I desire to prioritize strength, I incorporate exercises within the range of four to six repetitions. Nevertheless, this is discretionary and likely suboptimal for a strict hypertrophy regimen. As previously mentioned, engaging in low-repetition sets might necessitate performing a greater number of sets in order to achieve an equivalent level of muscular hypertrophy as moderate-repetition sets, which could potentially be unsustainable. I would like to propose the idea of exploring strength training at a later juncture and gradually reducing the intensity of your training phase, or adopting a combination of training approaches. This approach enables you to simultaneously enhance both strength and size.

Chapter Summary

The level of intensity is determined by the amount of weight placed on the bar relative to your maximum lifting capacity.

For the purpose of promoting hypertrophy, it is deemed optimal to adhere to an intensity range of approximately 60% to 85%, which corresponds to performing five to 20 repetitions per hard set.

Novice individuals are advised to initiate their heavier exercises in the moderate repetition range of approximately 8 to 12 in order to acquire the necessary skills for performing technically challenging barbell movements safely, while ensuring they do not approach failure too closely.

As a general principle, it is recommended that a significant majority, specifically around two-thirds to three-quarters, of the total weekly sets allocated for each major muscle group should consist of heavy or moderate intensity, with the remaining portion falling within the lighter range.

Focus predominantly on higher repetition ranges when targeting the smaller muscle groups.

It is recommended that your exercise regimen commences with high-intensity (compound) exercises and concludes with low-intensity (isolation) exercises.

Relative Effort

All right. The requisite aspects of volume, frequency, and intensity have been established, and you have already surveyed several commendable exercise routines. From a technical standpoint, it is possible that you have already created your initial program! Consequently, there are no obstacles remaining between you and the benefits you seek, am I correct?

If that task were to be accomplished with such simplicity, one would observe a greater prevalence of individuals exhibiting a notably muscular physique. It is possible to still make significant mistakes, even if the previous four steps were meticulously followed.

Please prepare yourself as we are about to discuss the final gap in our programming component - the concept of relative effort or training difficulty. It is imperative that we ascertain the optimal intensity level and perceived exertion of your workouts in order to achieve significant improvements. Maintain a vigilant lookout, for this is the domain where individuals often err egregiously, apart from matters of consistency.

It is observed that a significant number of weightlifters hold the misconception that they exert sufficient effort during their training sessions, though this is not the case. If, at any point during a workout, you have elected to prematurely conclude a set solely based on achieving a predetermined number of repetitions, it is plausible that you have also been culpable of this behavior. Alternatively, if you have ceased your sets due to perceiving them as challenging, despite having the potential to perform five or more additional repetitions if sufficiently motivated or compelled.

In my observation, this appears to be the predominant approach employed by the majority of individuals, which, in my opinion, is regrettable as it does not capitalize on the potential for significant muscular growth that can be achieved by pushing oneself close to the point of muscular failure during each set. This is the intended interpretation whenever I refer to a "hard set" — a set performed with high intensity until close to failure. Now, that prompts a series of inquiries, such as "To what degree must one exert oneself?" "How does one precisely gauge the level of intensity?" "Is it advisable to reach complete exhaustion in each set?" "Is it permissible to retain a few remaining repetitions?" "If so, what is the optimal number?" "And what considerations should be made for varying exercises?

Fortunately, a substantial body of research exists that provides us with ample evidence to confidently address these questions. Initially, in order to assess the level of exertion comparatively, one may utilize RIR (Repetitions in Reserve), which refers to the subjective evaluation of the number of repetitions remaining in one's capacity after concluding a set. For example:

Upon completing your final repetition, you speculate that you might have been capable of performing at most two additional repetitions.

1 repetition in reserve: Upon completing your last repetition, you believe that you could have potentially performed one additional repetition at maximum effort.

Upon completing your last repetition, you carefully return the barbell to its rack and recognize that you have reached your limit, rendering any additional repetitions unattainable.

Failure: Upon reaching the culmination of a physically demanding repetition, you proceed to attempt another one, only to be unsuccessful.

According to research findings, it has been indicated that the optimal range for muscle growth initiation begins at approximately 4 reps in reserve (RIR). Nevertheless, similar to the concept of volume, the principle of diminishing returns is equally applicable. Therefore, as you approach failure during each repetition, the subsequent muscle-building advantages diminish.

A measure of respiration rate reduction, amounting to 3 RIR, is significantly superior to that of 4.

Two repetitions in reserve (RIR) surpasses three in terms of efficacy.

Upon comparison, it can be observed that 1 RIR demonstrates a slight superiority over 2.

A rating of zero RIR is slightly superior to a rating of one.

Nonachievement is only marginally superior to a complete absence of results in terms of RIR.

Given that I am able to envision you pondering with confusion and contemplating, "Alright, the advantages of reaching the point of failure may indeed be insignificant." However, would it not be prudent to purposefully incur failure in the majority of my sets in order to optimize my muscle growth? Though the benefits may be modest in scale, they are nonetheless benefits, thus...."

I hear you. Upon initial observation, your inference would indeed be accurate. Nevertheless, it is imperative that you take into account additional factors during the course of your training. In this case:

Fatigue and injury risk.

Although the practice of performing sets to failure provides a more effective stimulus, it also results in considerably higher levels of fatigue in comparison to moderately challenging sets, particularly when performing compound exercises with significant loads. Consequently, this fatigue can have a detrimental impact on subsequent sets or sessions, consequently hindering potential progress in the future.

Envision engaging in a series of squats until reaching the point of complete muscular exhaustion. You diligently perform a final repetition, requiring approximately 12 seconds to complete. Despite being aware of your limitations, you still choose to proceed with this endeavor. Upon descending into the excavated opening, you exert your final reserves of energy in an attempt to rise upright for an additional duration of ten seconds, mindful of avoiding any spinal strain. Eventually, you are compelled to release the weighted bar onto the designated support structure, while ardently endeavoring to maintain bodily composure and emotional fortitude.

I am uncertain of your perspective, but in my own experience, I found it impossible to complete another productive set following this difficult experience, regardless of subsequent circumstances.

Certainly, squats serve as an exceptional instance (note: it is strongly advised to avoid reaching muscular failure during squat training sessions!). However, the approach might vary when considering an exercise such as a set of curls. Isolation exercises, in general, are characterized by being considerably easier to recuperate from. Therefore, they are more apt for being executed to the point of failure on a more frequent basis. However, it is unlikely that engaging in intense leg exercises or upper body compound movements would be suitable. Furthermore, it should be noted that work capacity, recovery ability, and pain tolerance also contribute to the situation at hand. Certain individuals may possess the capacity to repeatedly approach the brink of exhaustion without experiencing notable repercussions, even in activities such as the leg press. Others, including myself, may not possess the same ability and consequently endure a prolonged recovery period.

Furthermore, it is imperative to consistently bear in mind the potential risks associated with opting to push a set to the point of failure. There are several exercises that are not appropriate for it, as they may potentially place you, your joints, or your back in a compromised position, such as:

Barbell squat and the majority of its variations

Barbell bench press

Dumbbell flys

Dumbbell pull-overs

What is the overarching conclusion or lesson to be drawn from this? What level of training intensity is recommended for you?

It is advisable to engage in rigorous training that ensures substantial progress, while also being cautious not to excessively strain oneself to the point of jeopardizing future improvements.

If you are still a novice, this likely entails investing a reasonable amount of effort into each of your sets. Certainly, you may consider implementing the Recommended Repetitions in Reserve (RIR) approach outlined earlier, aiming to maintain an average RIR of one to two for most isolation exercises and three for most compound exercises throughout your training routine. However, it is probable that simply remembering to approach failure, exerting maximum effort during sets, and attempting to steadily improve your lifts may suffice. Rather than becoming excessively engrossed in it, it would be advisable to bear in mind this RIR method in order to maintain integrity. It is not a precise scientific discipline, in any case.

The majority of individuals tend to underestimate their Reserve Interest Rate (RIR), irrespective of the excessive attention they devote to it. Therefore, an individual may believe that they had three remaining repetitions in reserve, whereas they could have exerted themselves to complete an additional six repetitions at the very least.

Thus, what measures do you employ to guarantee a high level of endeavor without unnecessarily complicating matters? It is advisable to adhere to a moderate pace when repeating information. Based on my prior experiences, I have observed that the initial occurrence of decreased speed in execution typically transpires when the individual is approximately three to four repetitions away from reaching muscular fatigue. The initial repetition that begins to pose difficulty typically occurs approximately five to six repetitions from the current point. While it might appear trivial, an alternative approach would involve utilizing your facial expressions as an indicator to gauge the level of difficulty of your sets. If one does not exhibit a discernible facial expression or clench one's teeth, it is unlikely to be the case. Interesting fact: Each time I commence a fresh training cycle subsequent to a period of rest and recuperation, I experience facial discomfort as a result.

As previously mentioned, the RIR concept possesses certain limitations and is greatly influenced by one's attitude, experience, and present circumstances. Contrast the experience of attempting to train suboptimally after a night spent socializing with friends and lacking any motivation, with that of engaging in a workout session fueled by pre-workout supplementation subsequent to being provoked by someone during the commute to the gym.

Nonetheless, it can serve as a valuable instrument that facilitates the evaluation of the intensity of your sessions to ensure their optimal productivity. This becomes particularly advantageous as you progress in your training and develop a system to establish consistent standards for various exercises (e.g., 2 RIR corresponds to a certain level of exertion during bench presses, while 1 RIR represents a similar sensation during lat pull-downs, etc.).

If you fully embrace the forthcoming expansion guidelines, RIR may even be resolved through a self-solving mechanism. If one were to commence their program with an initial resistance-to-repetition ratio (RIR) of, for instance, 3, and consistently augment the weight or repetitions, it can be anticipated that they would progressively approach exhaustion over the subsequent weeks, unless possessing extraordinary strength akin to that of Superman.

However, in conclusion, I would like to reiterate: It is imperative to refrain from undertaking inadequate training efforts. Provide your RIR with the most accurate estimation and exert utmost dedication to your workouts, and you will achieve desired outcomes. Alternatively, failure to do so may result in a squandering of your valuable time.

Chapter Summary

Relative effort refers to the proximity to failure achieved in each of your working sets. It is quantified through the utilization of RIR (repetitions in reserve), which represents one's estimated remaining repetitions upon completion of one's sets.

Strive to achieve a Reps in Reserve (RIR) of no less than two or three in a majority of your sets in order to enhance optimal hypertrophy.

However, the majority of novices will be adequately served by prioritizing their utmost dedication to each set and temporarily keeping the concept of Reps in Reserve (RIR) in mind.

Exercising at an excessively low intensity level can lead to a significant increase in workload, resulting in highly inefficient or even completely ineffective training.

Excessive training, frequently pushing oneself to the point of failure, can result in significant fatigue, provide limited hypertrophic advantages, and potentially increase the likelihood of sustaining injuries.

Based on the specific muscle groups and exercises involved, it may be possible to engage in more frequent training to failure. This is particularly true for smaller muscle groups and isolation exercises that do not place you in a vulnerable position once you reach the point of failure.

It is imperative to ensure diligent training that yields favorable gains without jeopardizing future progress.

Commence your programs at approximately 2 repetitions in reserve (RIR) on average (subject to variation depending on the exercise); as you progressively elevate the intensity and/or repetitions in your program, your RIR will inherently reduce.

The Most Effective Exercises For Each Body Part To Stimulate Massive Amounts Of Muscle Growth

Chest

The pectoral muscles are often prioritized in male physique development due to their commonly perceived underdeveloped state in men. The considerable enthusiasm surrounding the phenomenon of "Chest Mondays" serves as tangible evidence of this claim. Engaging the pectoral muscles can pose a challenge, particularly during bench press exercises, as improper form may result in an excessive burden on the shoulders and triceps. As previously mentioned, a key aspect of weight training lies in the ability to perceive the stretching and contracting sensations within the targeted muscle group that one wishes to activate. If one does not experience the sensation of stretching and contracting the muscle, it indicates a lack of effectiveness in the workout, rendering it a futile use of time.

Presented herein are the sole exercises that would effectively aid in the development of pronounced pectoral muscles (with no occurrence of enlarged breast tissue, gentlemen):

The incline press exercise focuses on developing the upper pectoral muscles, frontal deltoids, and triceps.

The Flat Bench Press exercise is designed to engage and develop the pectoral muscles, alongside the front deltoids and triceps.

Chest Fly - A chest isolation exercise that eliminates the involvement of the triceps and exclusively targets the chest muscles, thereby directing all the tension towards the chest.

Pushups – Comparable to the Flat press exercise. Highly effective for establishing a profound cognitive-physical correlation with the pectoral muscles, as one can genuinely perceive an intensified hemodynamic response localized in the chest region while performing push-ups. To increase tension on the chest, engage in a wide grip push up while slightly rotating your hands in a clockwise direction.

Dips are a compound exercise that effectively target the pectoral muscles, triceps, and anterior deltoids. Ensure that you incorporate a slight forward inclination into your dipping motion to effectively engage your pectoral muscles. Should your posture remain upright during the dip, it is likely that you are primarily engaging your triceps.

These particular exercises are sufficient for attaining substantial muscular development in your chest. Please bear in mind that the "mind-muscle" connection is not merely a frivolous term that Arnold employed for the sake of sounding impressive. It is imperative to place substantial attention towards the extension and contraction of the chest during the performance of these exercises.

Back

The development of the back muscles presents a significant challenge, particularly for novices in the field of weight training. I vividly recall the initial stages of my weight training journey, where the adequate stimulation of my back muscles seemed elusive. When engaging in these exercises, it is imperative to ensure that the resistance is primarily felt by your back muscles rather than your arms. You can expect the muscles in your biceps and forearms to experience a sensation of increased blood flow, commonly referred to as a pump, which is a normal and inherent occurrence. However, I would encourage you to place significant emphasis on utilizing your back muscles to execute the movement of the weight.

Barbell Rows- Enhances the development of the musculature in the upper back region, while actively stimulating the involvement of the stabilizer muscles. I propose assuming a position atop a raised platform during the execution of barbell rows, whereby your body attains a parallel alignment with the ground, thus enabling a concentrated emphasis on the development of back musculature.

Dumbbell Rows – These exercises follow a similar concept to barbell rows. Aids in the development of both back thickness and lat muscles, while utilizing dumbbells to enhance the sensation of the stretching and flexing involved in the exercise.

Deadlifts- Effectively engage the lower body and back muscles. Exert a deliberate effort to firmly contract your shoulder blades, thereby extending your chest, in order to enhance the stimulation of your back muscles. WARNING: Engaging in this activity without proper posture may result in physical harm and potential injury. It is advised to begin with a lighter intensity and gradually progress to ensure proper technique and safety.

Pull-ups represent a timeless exercise effectively targeting the muscles of the back. Primarily focuses on the Latissimus dorsi, the muscular group that was renowned for its development in Bruce Lee. Furthermore, it promotes the activation of the forearms and biceps.

The activation of the back muscles can pose considerable challenges for individuals who are new to exercise. Therefore, instead of immediately attempting a 220 pound deadlift, it is advisable to commence with lighter weights and actively concentrate on engaging the back muscles throughout each exercise. Once you have developed proficiency in engaging your back muscles through these exercises, proceed to increase the weight load.

Shoulders

The muscle that I derive the most personal satisfaction from training. When engaging in shoulder training, it is crucial to bear in mind that the shoulder is composed of three distinct components, namely the front deltoid, side deltoid, and rear deltoids. These exercises are designed to effectively stimulate each individual deltoid head, contributing to the attainment of a well-defined V-taper physique.

The Military Press focuses on engaging the different regions of the deltoid muscles along with the triceps. I would propose that you engage in this activity while in an upright position, as it will not only enhance your core strength but also engage a greater number of stabilizer muscles.

Front Raises - This exercise specifically focuses on the front deltoid muscle. Maintain proper form and aim to control your body movement, avoiding excessive swinging.

Lateral Raises - specifically focus on activating the lateral deltoid muscles, thereby contributing to the attainment of a pronounced v-taper silhouette that accentuates broad shoulders. It is essential to bear in mind that the sensation of resistance should be specifically felt in the side deltoid muscle, while minimizing any movement in the trapezius muscle.

Engage in Deltoid raises, with a specific focus on the rear delts, in order to enhance the prominence of your shoulders and create a more pronounced three-dimensional effect from the back. Moreover, it contributes to the enhancement of your posture. It is a commonly observed phenomenon that individuals often possess well-developed front deltoids but lack proper development in their rear deltoids. This imbalance results in an aesthetically displeasing gait and posture irregularities.

Dumbbell Shoulder Presses—Similar to the military press, this exercise allows you to identify potential muscular disparities and additionally enhances the extent of stretch and flexion in the motion.

The Clean and Press focuses on the lower extremities during the cleaning phase, making it an exceptional compound exercise for enhancing overall muscular size and strength. WARNING: It is essential to exercise caution as this particular activity has the potential to compromise your physical posture if performed without due care. To mitigate any risks, it is advised to initiate the exercise with lighter intensity and gradually progress.

Legs

The "no-show muscles". The muscles that are typically not favored by 99% of individuals frequenting the gym, yet necessitate their attention and training. The lower body constitutes half of your physique; therefore, it is imperative to engage in rigorous training for optimal enhancement of functional strength and to avoid any imbalances that may arise from a disproportionate upper body and underdeveloped lower limbs, resulting in an incongruous, skeletal appearance.

Squats -Of Course. The ultimate monarch of lower body workouts. Effectively engages and strengthens the muscles of your lower body, particularly emphasizing the glutes. WARNING: Exercise extreme caution with regard to this matter as well. When performing this movement, you will be required to handle substantial weight. Although heavy loads can lead to significant improvements, they also pose a risk of severe injury if precautions are not taken.

Front Squats - A comprehensive lower body exercise that primarily targets the quadriceps while also engaging the stabilizer muscles. It may require a significant amount of time to achieve proficiency in executing the correct form for this exercise, thus it is advisable to initiate the regimen with minimal weight and gradually increase the intensity.

Lunges are a comprehensive lower body exercise that primarily targets the quadriceps. This task can be performed using either barbells or dumbbells. When utilizing dumbbells, one may experience a degree of strain in the forearm region, an occurrence that can yield either advantageous or disadvantageous outcomes depending on one's objectives.

Power Cleans are a highly effective exercise that facilitates the development of strength and promotes the capacity to exert increased force on the leg muscles. An additional Olympic lifting exercise that has the potential to significantly enhance muscle growth. The task may present challenges, hence it is advisable to begin with minimal intensity and gradually increase.

The straight legged deadlift is an excellent exercise for developing strength, particularly focusing on the hamstring muscles. Another exercise that can pose significant risks if your form is imprecise, hence it is advisable to commence with lighter weights and progress gradually.

Calf Raises – One may opt for the utilization of a machine or alternatively employ a barbell or dumbbells while performing calf raises on an elevated platform. My calves are a specific area of vulnerability for me, which necessitates consistent and focused muscle training. Direct your attention towards the stretching and flexing of the calf muscles, and undoubtedly, they will flourish.

Biceps

The sole means of impressing a refined woman is by presenting her with a pair of tickets to the firearms exhibition... "and determine whether or not she approves of the merchandise." - Ron Burgundy. Personally, I find that my biceps are considerably underdeveloped, necessitating rigorous training to ensure harmonious proportions with the remainder of my physique. It is worth emphasizing that the biceps are also engaged during numerous back exercises. Nevertheless, provided below are several isolation exercises that can be employed to augment bicep activation and promote their muscular development.

Standing Barbell Curls - Undoubtedly, this exercise holds a prominent place in Arnold's list of preferred bicep workouts. Ensure that you are achieving the appropriate muscular contraction at the zenith of the exercise and experiencing the necessary elongation at the nadir. Furthermore, make an effort to minimize the oscillation of the body. When performing cheat curls, it is permissible to exhibit slight swinging movements. Conversely, during standard barbell curls, it is advised to minimize any traces of swinging.

Incorporating Incline Dumbbell Curls facilitates a heightened degree of extension at the lower end of the exercise owing to the inclined posture provided by the bench.

Concentration Curls - Place particular emphasis on the contraction of the biceps at the peak of the curl. This activity can be accomplished in either a seated position or by assuming a bent-over posture.

Triceps

Enhancing the triceps muscles will not solely enhance your proficiency in pressing exercises such as the bench press, military press, and dumbbell presses, but it will also contribute to significant arm muscle development, considering that the triceps constitute two-thirds of the arm. The triceps experience significant stimulation during exercises involving pressing movements. Nevertheless, here are some impressive isolation exercises that can be employed to enhance their development.

The close grip bench press is highly effective for achieving tricep overload. Please ensure that you maintain an appropriate distance between your grip and the object to avoid any potential harm to your wrists.

Dumbbell Skull crushers are an excellent exercise for precisely targeting the long head of the tricep and achieving a thorough contraction. Ensure that you maintain a consistent level of tension in the triceps throughout the execution of this exercise, avoiding any transfer of resistance from the triceps to the shoulders. The activity can be performed in a standing or seated position - standing engages additional stabilizer muscles and stimulates the core, while sitting allows for increased tricep isolation.

Core

Indeed, should you desire to attain a well-defined abdominal region, it is imperative to engage in specific exercises targeting the abdominal muscles. It is imperative to acknowledge that the presence of well-developed abdominal muscles alone is insufficient for their visibility if one's body fat percentage exceeds a certain level. Presented below are a selection of abdominal exercises designed to enhance your core strength.

Prone Hold. A straightforward and uncomplicated workout routine dedicated to enhancing the strength of your core.

Cross Body Crunch - The exercise consistently utilized by pugilists. Focuses on your abdominal muscles, particularly the obliques.

Leg Raises – A highly effective exercise for engaging and strengthening the muscles in your lower abdominal region. Typically, I perform these tasks in a supine position on the ground.

Sit-ups - Yet another enduring exercise that has withstood the trials of time.

From my perspective, it would be advisable to refrain from placing excessive emphasis on the abdominal muscles. These muscles are relatively small in size and function independently without significant involvement of other muscle groups, which limits the release of growth hormone required for maximal muscle development and significant improvements in size. As an individual, I exclusively engage in a brief 4-minute series of abdominal exercises subsequent to each workout. Nevertheless, if you are inclined to devote 30 minutes to abdominal training, feel free to do so without restraint.

Takeaways

These are the most effective exercises that will provide optimal results. If you were to invest your resources primarily in a select few of these exercises, opt for the heavy compound lifts. The exercises encompassed within this category include the bench press, military press, deadlifts, clean and press, rows, and several others. The compound lifts are the sole exercises requisite for developing an exceptional physique, fostering substantial gains in muscle mass, size, and power.

The underlying biology

As previously stated, many women experience apprehension in regard to engaging in weightlifting exercises due to their aversion to developing excessive muscle mass. You will be pleased to learn that your female physique is inherently ill-suited for substantial muscle gain as per biological factors. However, engaging in weightlifting activities results in the gradual augmentation of your lean muscle mass. Having a higher proportion of lean muscle mass facilitates a greater capacity for fat metabolism, even during periods of physical inactivity. This combination allows for enhanced fat burning in the body, thereby preventing the development of excessive muscle mass.

If that rationale fails to persuade you that weightlifting does not lead to a bulky physique, consider placing deliberation on the impact of your hormones. Females exhibit insufficient testosterone levels to achieve significant muscle hypertrophy. Furthermore, a significant proportion of females fail to consume an adequate amount of calories necessary to support the development and maintenance of robust muscle mass. Contrary to popular fallacies, solely engaging in weightlifting will not result in the automatic growth of larger muscles. As previously stated in the preceding chapter, it is essential to consume food in order to provide energy for one's body. Those individuals who assert themselves as being muscular are either envisioning the outcome or making dramatic alterations to their dietary habits.

Now that we have addressed that matter, let us now focus on the crucial aspect of bodybuilding: your body type! As previously mentioned, every individual here possesses unique physical attributes. Could you please elaborate on your personality type and describe the steps you take to achieve your highest potential? That is precisely the purpose of our presence. Please proceed to learn about your individual type and the corresponding macronutrient ratios most suitable for you.

Different body types
Ectomorph
We would like to initiate by emphasizing that these descriptions may not entirely align with every individual. Although it is possible to select most of one's characteristics, it is common for individuals to possess a combination of traits. It is crucial to identify the specific major type that closely aligns with your characteristics, in order to customize your nutrition and exercise plan accordingly. We shall commence with the most diminutive among the physical constitutions.

If you possess an ectomorphic physique, it is probable that your body type would be reminiscent of that of a competitive long-distance runner. It is likely that you possess a more petite skeletal structure, smaller extremities, and a heightened metabolic rate, which results in a more slender physique. A considerably elevated metabolic rate implies that you possess the advantageous ability of your body to effectively process a higher quantity of carbohydrates. In terms of the proportion of macronutrients, we recommend adhering to a ratio of 50 percent carbohydrates, 30 percent protein, and 20 percent fat.

Mesomorph

If an individual is classified as a mesomorph, their physical appearance typically resembles that of a gymnast or a bodybuilder. This specific body type provides an optimal basis for muscular development, as it possesses a harmonious capacity for maintaining leanness while simultaneously acquiring muscle mass. This somatotype exhibits a moderate-sized skeletal framework and is expected to display a predominantly athletic physique. If you perceive yourself as possessing this physique, it is advisable to adhere to a macronutrient distribution resembling a proportion of approximately 40 percent carbohydrates, 30 percent protein, and 30 percent fat. In contrast to individuals with an ectomorphic physique, your body exhibits a reduced tolerance for carbohydrates. Instead, nourish your body with protein to facilitate the development of muscle!

Endomorph

Conversely, there exist individuals who possess an endomorph body constitution. These women bear a semblance to powerlifters, more or less. Given their significant bone structure, it should be noted that they possess a considerable physical size and strength in comparison to the majority. Given their physique, individuals with this body type may find it more beneficial to adopt a dietary regimen characterized by a higher inclusion of healthy fats and a reduced intake of carbohydrates. The optimal distribution of macronutrients for individuals of this body type is comprised of 25 percent carbohydrates, 35 percent protein, and 40 percent fat, as suggested.

As evident from the evidence presented, there exists a compelling rationale for the non-universal applicability of a singular dietary regimen. Once you have determined the body type that closely aligns with your physiological characteristics, you may commence the process of formulating a dietary plan accordingly. Evidently, individual bodies require varying types of nutrients. Ultimately, your primary emphasis should be on incorporating high-quality culinary ingredients to yield superior outcomes. We would advise preparing your own meals in order to adhere more closely to the proposed regimen. If you choose to venture outside, it is advisable to bear in mind your dietary goals in order to stay aligned with them.

Having acquainted yourself with the necessary nutrients essential for your body and its unique requirements, let us now proceed to the segment dedicated to the acquisition of appropriate equipment. Similar to how your dietary habits may vary, the selection of bodybuilding equipment can also differ based on the specific objectives you aim to achieve. Proceed with the exploration to discern the optimal regimen that will yield favorable outcomes for your individual needs!

What is the recommended frequency of exercise for a bodybuilder aiming to achieve muscle gains?

Achieving the appropriate equilibrium between strength training and cardiovascular exercise is crucial when it comes to developing lean muscles. Engaging in excessive activity carries the risk of overtraining, potentially resulting in the loss of your hard-earned muscle. However, should you fail to elevate your performance and dedicate sufficient effort, your progress in muscle development will be negligible.

Cardiovascular exercise

Adhere to incorporating several days of cardiovascular exercise into your weekly routine, focusing on shorter, more intense sessions such as 25 minutes of High-Intensity Interval Training (HIIT).

Strength exercise

It is recommended that you engage in weight training at least three times per week. According to a study, the act of engaging in physical labor for a minimum of two days per week is anticipated to positively impact and enhance muscle growth and development. The manner in which you organize your exercises and the duration of time you dedicate to strength training is contingent upon your current level of fitness.

Presented here are several foundational principles of strength training that you may consider incorporating into your routine, accompanied by a exemplifying exercise.

Please consider undertaking this timetable, taking into account your level of expertise.

Novice: Engage in strength training sessions (comprising full-body exercises) for two to three days on a weekly basis.

Intermediate: Consistently engage in strength training sessions lasting three to four days per week. Divide the exercise routine according to the specific focus on either the upper body, lower body, or individual body parts.

Advanced: For those at an elevated fitness level, it is recommended to engage in strength training for a duration of four to five days per week. Additionally, individuals who possess exceptional physical conditioning may consider organizing their weekly workout routine to consist of three consecutive training days followed by a single rest day.

If adhering to a four-day strength training regimen resonates with you, it may be advisable to divide your week into discrete segments, focusing on lower body (legs) and upper body (arms, chest, and abs) exercises. For instance:

Monday: Focusing on the musculature of the upper half of the body.

Tuesday: Focusing on the lower extremities

Wednesday: Opportunities for relaxation or cardiovascular exercise.

Thursday: Focused on the upper extremities.

Friday: Focusing on the lower extremities

Saturday: Engage in either relaxation or cardiovascular exercise.

Sunday: Dedicate to leisure or engage in cardiovascular activities

It is comprehensible that you may perceive your muscle growth progress to be slower than anticipated. The potential hurdle you may encounter is known as "the formidable plateau."

When you consistently engage the same muscle groups in repetitive exercises with a consistent intensity over an extended duration, there is a high probability that your body will cease to exhibit any further response.

In order to transition back to a stage of muscle development, it is necessary to introduce variations into your regimen. Herein lie several discrete approaches to accomplish this task.

•Increase the resistance when performing weightlifting exercises.

• Transition to a workout regimen that is distinct from your current one.

• Modify the quantity of repetitions and sets being executed. • Adjust the number of repetitions and sets that you are currently undertaking. • Alter the count of reps and sets being performed. • Revise the number of repetitions and sets you are engaging in. By varying the range of repetitions, you integrate lighter and heavier loads to elicit more substantial advancements in strength and muscular development. As an example, a substantial session will consist of a range of 3 to 5 repetitions, a moderate session will encompass a range of 8 to 12 repetitions, and a gentle session will entail a range of 15 to 20 repetitions.

In regards to enhancing the strength of your competitive advantage, it is imperative to ensure that you allocate ample time for your body to recuperate in between sessions of strength training. Engaging in similar behaviors, sustaining a high level of physical exertion for an extended duration may impede the process of recuperation and result in long-term muscle loss.

If managing the implementation of regular days off every week proves challenging, you may want to conceive of these days as periods of active rejuvenation. Engage in a gentle yoga session or allocate more time for stretching exercises.

www.ingramcontent.com/pod-product-compliance
Lightning Source LLC
Chambersburg PA
CBHW051734020426
42333CB00014B/1296